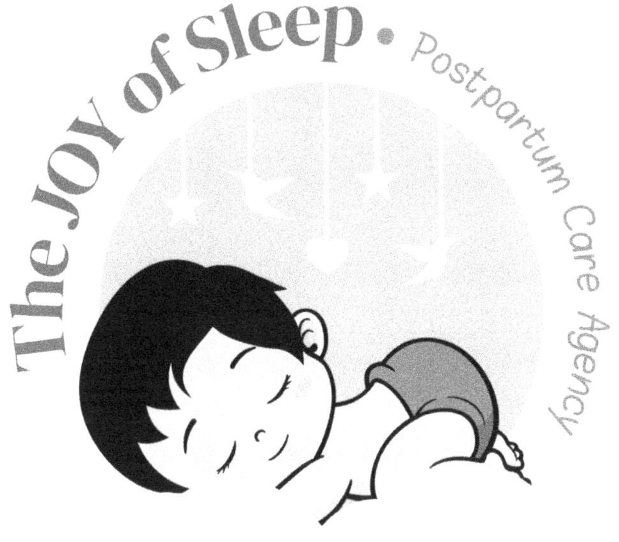

Newborn Care Specialist

Training Manual

Joy Bostrom

ISBN: 9798869151216

Some information in this manual is taken directly from other sources. I would also like to thank all of my colleagues who shared their ideas and suggestions.

Note that some of the information presented here is from researchers and specialists. However, there are times when the information reflects personal opinions from experience.

This manual is for reference only. Use this information to supplement the advice from the baby's physician or qualified health provider. This book is not a substitute for consultations with your health care provider, medical investigation, or treatment. Exercise discretion when advising clients on newborn care.

The author has tried to ensure accuracy and timeliness but assumes no liability for warranties, expressed or implied, regarding the accuracy or reliability of the information.

Contents

Introduction

What is a Newborn Care Specialist?

Introducing a newborn into the world is a transformative, challenging experience, particularly at night. Sleepless nights, constant feedings, and adjusting to a new family dynamic can overwhelm parents. To address these challenges, professionals have emerged to help during the postpartum period. This section discusses the different types of infant caregivers and how being a Newborn Care Specialist differs from the others.

A Newborn Care Specialist (NCS) helps parents with their newborns, typically at night. They are professionals who have in-depth training and knowledge. They usually work 8-10 hours overnight but can also work 24-hour shifts or during the day. The main job of an NCS is to take care of the newborn, ensuring their needs are met while the parents have a chance to rest. They also teach parents about caring for the baby, including basic care, swaddling, self-soothing, routines and schedules, and sleep training strategies.

Newborn Care Specialists stay up-to-date on research with the latest guidelines and recommendations and have advanced education on how to address various issues and challenges that can occur with newborns.

Glossary

- **Doula:** an experienced person who provides non-medical support during childbirth and postpartum with a perspective that encompasses the entire family. She will be helping the mom, the other parent, siblings, and extended family to integrate the new addition to the family experience. A "Birth Doula" helps during labor, and a "Postpartum Doula" helps after the birth. Postpartum doulas are not typically trained in sleep conditioning for newborns, although they are an extra hand who can help the new parents.
- **Nanny or Night Nanny:** a person caring for children in someone else's home; typically not professionally trained.

- **Night Nurse:** a professionally trained RN or LVN who helps and educates new moms about newborn care. Night nurses often help with premature newborn care because of the infant's specialized needs, like apnea monitoring, G-tube, or trachea care.
- **Newborn Care Specialist (NCS):** a non-medical person trained and specializing in baby care. While a Doula's primary focus is on the mother's well-being, an NCS focuses on the newborn and educating the parents on newborn issues.
- **Mother's Helper:** assists with childcare but isn't trained in newborn care.
- **Wet Nurse:** a term used for centuries for a person who breastfeeds a newborn for a mother who can't or doesn't want to. Formula use has mostly replaced wet nursing.

NCS Responsibilities

A Newborn Care Specialist's responsibilities vary depending on their work shift and the parents' requirements. Among the duties they will provide:

- educate and support parents
- help with a smooth transition to having a newborn
- troubleshoot issues
- maintain feeding and sleep logs
- assist with breastfeeding
- soothe babies
- perform tasks like diapering, dressing, bottle preparation, bathing, circumcision care, umbilical cord care
- establish feeding schedules
- help with sleep training

Some Newborn Care Specialists assist with sleep training beyond three months, handle reflux, work with multiples, and care for premature babies. These specialists have experience in these areas and are uniquely skilled to assist.

The Importance of Maintaining a Feeding and Sleep Log

Maintaining a log at work for each baby is a critical part of an NCS's job. The log acts as a crucial map, providing vital information to detect any abnormalities. Also, when working as a team, it's essential for the next person to review the patterns. This includes details like the number of wet diapers, bowel movements, total ounces consumed, feeds, sleep patterns, and signs of colic.

These notes are crucial for parents, ourselves, and for liability reasons. If there are signs of reflux or a baby is making sour faces, we document it and provide informed suggestions or guide them to seek answers. For instance, if a baby shows a pattern of no wet diapers, it could indicate various issues like insufficient milk, hunger, dietary changes needed, or a reaction to a vaccine. Any unusual occurrences, such as bright orange or pink urine, should be documented.

In addition to keeping track of the numbers, writing down observations and communicating them accurately to parents is also important. While you may inform parents verbally, writing it down ensures they remember and acknowledges your professional communication.

Analyzing patterns and information is crucial. Understanding the value of written information helps interpret the situation effectively. Always seek clarification from others if unsure, be it another NCS or the parents. Being an intuitive caregiver involves examining the whole picture, including the baby's behavior, skin color, and eyes. As newborn care specialists, our role goes beyond babysitting; we are discerning and attentive professionals.

Compensation

Newborn Care Specialists earn hourly wages starting from $25, increasing based on experience, health issues, and the number of newborns. Rates range from $25-$50 per hour.

Work Schedule

Newborn Care Specialists set their schedule, usually working on a contractual basis for one week to three months. Weekly hours vary. Depending on client needs, they may work nights, days, or 24/7.

Work Location

Newborn Care Specialists usually work in clients' homes. Some may choose to travel to different states or cities to accept positions.

Newborn Care Specialist Interns

Newborn Care Specialist Interns have taken NCS training but lack experience. However, to get positions, they need experience. Several of the marketing suggestions discussed in this section are also avenues for gaining knowledge, such as joining parenting groups and networking. NCS Interns may shadow experienced Newborn Care Specialists, work as a paid helper, or gain experience through volunteer work.

Marketing Your Skill

Like any business, marketing is a must. For Newborn Care Specialists, there are different strategies, including:

- using agencies
- networking with friends who are Newborn Care Specialists
- relying on referrals (when your clients are happy, they will refer you to their friends and family)
- using online platforms
- advertising through various means, including newspaper ads, social media ads, brochures, business cards, etc.
- building a website
- joining parenting groups

Typical Night for an NCS

Newborn Care Specialists typically start between 7 pm and 10 pm. The routine is different, depending on the baby. An NCS will usually begin by discussing the baby with parents; this is baby-focused and not to discuss your personal issues. This nightly discussion about the baby may include educating them on any problems they are unaware of, taking sleep training steps, instructing them on bathing or other needs, or helping the mom organize her day. Then, the NCS will feed the baby if needed and then go to bed. An NCS will wake up when the baby does, soothe them back to sleep if necessary, and feed them if it's been more than three hours. Depending on the baby's sleep schedule, if the NCS can feed before they leave in the morning, the mother will have an extra three hours of sleep. NCSs have no responsibility for siblings, pets, or housework at night.

If the NCS is on a daytime schedule, they will be in charge of the baby's needs, including whatever the parents require concerning the newborn.

Why Parents Need NCSs

Parents are advised to sleep when the baby sleeps, but babies wake up frequently. Lack of continuous sleep can lead to sleep deprivation, affecting memory and mental health, and can lead to postpartum depression.

Section 1: The Infant Care Practitioner

Chapter 1: The Intuitive Caregiver

We will cover many beneficial qualities for a caregiver in this training manual. We will start with the essential trait needed to become a highly sought-after and effective infant care practitioner: intuition.

Listening to your intuition is relying on your innate impulses, inner wisdom, and heart to guide your decisions. Being connected with your intuition enables you to detect signs and react in a way that aligns with the needs of those you care for. Weaving intuition with clear communication allows you to create and maintain active yet subtle contact with the mother, baby, and family. Your intuition enhances decision-making, problem-solving, comfort, and support.

Deepening your use of intuition makes it easier to give clients compassionate care tailored to their individual needs. The great news is that intuition can be strengthened through repetition and introspection.

Intuition is the most crucial skill for this line of employment. Developing and employing your intuition will make you the region's best and most in-demand practitioner.

Additional essential qualities needed are the capacity to love and care. These three traits are interwoven; you must be in tune with all three to be your best for this task.

Chapter 2: Energetic Hygiene

Awareness of your energetic hygiene is crucial for developing intuition, especially for caregivers. Energetic hygiene involves staying mindful of your energy, the energy in your surroundings, and that of others. It's not just about awareness; you must also learn to control your energy. Unwinding before caregiving, leaving emotional baggage behind, and staying focused on the task enhance caregiver presence. Kindness, adaptability, and spontaneity contribute to maintaining and strengthening this presence.

Babies and parents are sensitive to the energy and emotions around them. Caregivers need to be attentive to the energy they project, control their thoughts, and be mindful of what they see or hear when they are with the infant. Considering the potential effects of electromagnetic fields (EMF) and wireless gadgets, such as cell phones, is also crucial for ensuring a safe environment for the infant.

Listening is another essential skill for caregivers. Allowing parents to express emotions without taking up all their time or interjecting personal experiences is important. Caregivers should avoid assuming parents want their input and focus on listening attentively, offering assistance as needed.

Various skills and traits, including compassion and effective communication, are necessary for caregivers. Providing the best care for the baby while fostering a positive environment requires these qualities. Combining intuitive connection, energetic hygiene, and compassionate care establishes a solid foundation for becoming a sought-after caregiver.

The following are energy tips you can use.

Mirror Calm

Reflecting calmness instead of joining parents' anxiety helps the infant and their parents feel safer. Consider your words carefully before speaking. Ask parents if they need help; don't assume you already know what they need.

Ask for Permission

Another essential aspect of excellent caregiving is asking for permission. Before making recommendations, do thorough research. Never assume anything. Double-check and explain what is anticipated or required to ensure everyone is on the same page.

Relax

Caretakers create a quiet and secure environment for infants and parents by maintaining composure. Speaking correctly, using uplifting phrases, and practicing harmony contribute to a pleasant and encouraging atmosphere.

Be Honest and Transparent

Openness, asking instead of assuming, being forceful yet gentle, and setting firm and kind boundaries are crucial caregiver traits. It's acceptable not to have all the answers, and seeking assistance or advice when needed is a sign of strength, not weakness.

Connect

Building trust and a good relationship with parents is facilitated by connecting with them and being present physically and emotionally. Talking to the infant and explaining what is happening and why fosters a sense of security and comfort.

Use Positive Visualization and Imagining

Cultivate a positive outlook and peace through positive visualization. Manage stress, encourage relaxation, and control emotions in difficult situations using techniques like breathing, closing eyes, humming, or tapping.

It's important to remember that infants are empathic and sense the feelings and thoughts of those around them. Create a sense of security and happiness by thinking positive thoughts, projecting optimism, and being present with your energy and attention.

Take Care of Your Health

When caring for a newborn, prioritize your physical and emotional health. Sleep and rest balance the emotional body and help you handle stress. Know when to intervene to help a baby or parent calm down and understand how to get out of fight or flight mode.

Examining potential long-term impacts and taking breaks from night shifts is vital due to the long-term effects of sleep deprivation. Caregivers should prioritize their rest.

Prioritizing self-care helps caregivers manage stress and provide the best care for the infant and their family. Some helpful self-care practices include:

- Creating a quiet and dark environment for naps or rest
- Engaging in relaxation techniques like massage or meditation

- Eating a healthy and balanced diet to support well-being
- Incorporating regular exercise into the routine
- Prioritizing sleep with a consistent schedule
- Engaging in joyful activities or spending time with loved ones
- Taking breaks or changing the scenery
- Playing and having fun to promote joy and playfulness

Chapter 3: Ethics for Newborn Care Professionals

Ethics for newborn care professionals are essential to ensuring that infants receive the best possible care. Newborn Care Specialists give babies and their families the most outstanding care possible by following specific moral guidelines. The following are ethical principles that newborn care professionals should keep in mind.

- **Respect for Autonomy:** Newborn care professionals should respect the right of parents to make decisions about their baby's care unless those decisions are likely to cause harm to the baby.
- **Beneficence:** Newborn care professionals should act in the baby's best interests, providing the highest quality care possible and taking steps to ensure the baby's well-being.
- **Do No Harm:** Newborn care professionals should not take actions that could cause physical or emotional harm to the baby.
- **Confidentiality:** Newborn care professionals should keep all information about the baby and their family confidential. Your position may depend on your ability to be discreet. Some clients may ask for a confidentiality agreement. The exceptions to this rule are where disclosure is required by law or necessary to protect the baby if there is abuse; in these cases, you are obligated to report it to the police or child protective services.
- **Informed Consent:** Parents should be fully advised about the risks and benefits of any techniques used to care for their baby and have the opportunity to ask questions to make informed decisions.
- **Cultural Sensitivity:** Newborn care professionals should respect the cultural and religious beliefs of the baby's family and should strive to provide culturally appropriate care.

- **Professionalism:** Newborn care professionals should always maintain high standards of professionalism and ethical conduct, including maintaining appropriate boundaries with clients and their families. Professionalism reassures parents and helps them trust you with the care of their infant.

Chapter 4: Interview Preparation

This section provides tips to prepare for an interview for an infant care position. Here are some things to consider:

- **Review the job description:** Ensure that you are familiar with the duties and requirements of the position so you can tailor your responses to the particular requirements of the role.
- **Display your Experience:** Be sure to highlight your experience with young children, whether from babysitting, volunteer work, or paid employment. Describe how your prior experiences have helped to prepare you for this job.
- **Prepare to Talk About Safety and Health Procedures:** Taking care of infants involves a great deal of responsibility for their safety and health, so be ready to talk about your knowledge and experience with techniques like CPR, first aid, and good cleanliness habits.
- **Showcase your Interpersonal Skills:** Working with infants requires patience, empathy, and the capacity for successful communication with parents and other caregivers. Be prepared to discuss how you acquired these abilities through prior experiences.
- **Demonstrate Your Flexibility:** Working with infants can be unpredictable, so showing that you're adaptable and flexible is critical. Prepare to talk about how you have dealt with unforeseen circumstances and how you may modify your plans and routines to suit the child's requirements better.
- **Always be truthful and respectful while discussing your experiences and credentials.** Ask questions if you have any doubts. Additionally, always respect the interviewer while being upbeat and eager to learn.

4.1 Interview Tips

Clients want an NCS who is experienced, responsible, and trustworthy because you'll be caring for their newborn. Here are some interview tips to help you reflect these principles.

- Confirm interview place and time 24 hours prior to meeting.
- Be on time.
- Know the way to the interview location to avoid being late or lost.
- Add 15 minutes to your travel time. If you arrive early, park nearby, review client information and prepare any additional questions.
- If you'll be more than 5 minutes late despite these steps, call and let them know. Confirm they still have time to meet with you.
- Prepare for the interview by anticipating questions and preparing concise answers.
- Clarify salary details if uncertain and make sure they understand your charges.
- Understand the job responsibilities to connect your skills and accomplishments to the position.
- Dress appropriately to show respect and make a good impression.
- Use proper speech without slang or improper grammar to communicate effectively.
- Maintain good eye contact to display confidence and avoid negative impressions.
- Guide the interview if needed, as some interviewers may not be skilled.
- Be clear about your career goals to avoid confusion about the offered position and salary.
- Ask well-thought-out questions to gain knowledge about the position's responsibilities, environment, and expectations.
- Have a good resume that lets you easily discuss your skills and experience.
- Turn off or silence your cell phone before entering the home.
- Learn the names of the family and use them when you refer to them in conversation.
- Demonstrate your knowledge by showing how to swaddle and asking to see the nursery. Discuss the support they will have from family and friends, feeding plans, and sleep training.
- Ask what their expectations are of you. Having this clear from the beginning will go a long way to having everyone happy with the results.

- Send a Thank You note after the interview. In the note, reference something you talked about in the interview.
- Compile a binder of information you can share about your previous work, contact information, reference letters, biography, and certificates. You can also include a background check, a recommended reading list, an example of how you record the newborn's schedule, a copy of an invoice, and a copy of your contract.

Chapter 5: On the Job

Newborn Care Specialists should use the following protocols while on the job:

- Ask permission before eating any of the client's food. Many clients like to provide snacks. Be respectful and conscientious. Bring your own snacks or food if you work the night shift.
- On-the-Job Hygiene: Use your own towel, clean up after you use the bathroom, and wash your hands after every use. Leave where you sleep as you found it. Remove shoes at the door and bring slippers or indoor shoes if needed. Wash hands regularly. If sick, ask the parents if they want you to come or wear a mask.
- Turn off your cell phone before entering. Set to vibrate if expecting a call. Don't talk or text in front of clients.
- Always ask for permission before using anything. If you use something in the middle of the night, inform the clients in the morning.
- Don't get personal. Focus on the baby and your job. Avoid asking for favors, accepting things, or hinting at needs. Don't use their equipment unless specified in your contract.
- Confirm duties and expectations on the first night. Leave on time, and communicate with clients about any household security system and how to enter and leave each shift.
- Problem-solving: Discuss any issues regarding the baby promptly. If it's about your work, meet with the parents to find a solution for everyone.
- We usually recommend bringing a change of clothes, toiletries, a pillow, warm layers (some houses are cold), and any other personal supplies you would like to have during your shift.

5.1 Appearance

Here are some general guidelines for dressing as a Newborn Care Specialist:

- **Comfortable clothing:** NCS work can involve long hours and physical activity, so wearing comfortable and practical attire is essential. Clothes should allow for full movement and not be too tight or restrictive. Scrubs in solid colors are recommended.
- **Neat and clean appearance:** Your clothing should be neat and clean, without holes or stains.
- **Avoid strong fragrances:** Newborns have sensitive skin and respiratory systems, so it's best to avoid wearing perfumes, colognes, or other scented products. No makeup is recommended; if necessary, keep it minimal. Personal hygiene is also essential, as you will be close to newborns; shower and put on unscented deodorant.
- **Dress modestly:** As an NCS, you will work in people's homes and should dress modestly and professionally. Avoid clothing that is too revealing or provocative.
- **Follow any specific guidelines from the family or agency:** Depending on the family or agency you work for, there may be particular dress code requirements or preferences. Always follow these guidelines to ensure you are meeting their expectations.
- **Hands and nails:** The appearance and cleanliness of your hands are important. It's vital to have short and natural nails. Long or fake nails are inappropriate for this line of work. It is also recommended to wear minimal, if any, hand jewelry, especially rings that could scratch the baby.

5.2 Leaving on Good Terms

At the end of your time with the newborn, it is beneficial to leave on excellent terms. One way to ensure this is to have an exit interview. Let them know how much you enjoyed their hospitality and your time with the baby and them. Inform them that you are available to answer any questions. An exit letter can be a great way to ask for a reference or letter of recommendation.

5.3 If Terms are Not Amicable

There may be times when something isn't clicking. Remember, parents often lack sleep, and mothers can have out-of-balance hormones. Things happen. We all learn from mistakes. However, if you are being "let go" frequently, you might look at what you are doing that is causing any issues.

Find compromises when possible, negotiate an amicable end, and ensure that the clients do not spread negative opinions with their contacts that can come back to haunt you.

Homework for Section 1

- Write a short introductory bio about yourself.
- Write an intention for your business.
- Write a personal mission statement for your business.
- Create a portfolio or binder and create a digital portfolio.
- With the information in this Chapter, how can I improve my current practices?
- What do I contribute positively to the family I work with?
- Optional: 10 goals (personal, professional, fun, and love) written in present voice; a statement about each goal.

Section 2: Getting to Know Baby

Chapter 6: What To Expect with a Healthy Newborn

Newborn babies have distinctive characteristics, which can indicate their health and well-being. A general, overall inspection of the newborn can be assessed with the guidelines in this section.

6.1 Size, Weight, and other Vitals

The following are average measurements and vital measurements for a healthy newborn according to the World Health Organization (WHO):

- Weight: 7lbs 6oz (3.35 kg) for males and 7lbs 2oz (3.23 kg) for females
- Length: 19 - 20in or 48.2 - 50.8cm
- Respiration of 30 breaths per minute and shallow.
- Rectal temperature of a newborn is 98.6° F (37° C). A normal temperature range can be between 96.8° F (36° C) and 100.3° F (37.9° C).
- Resting heart rate for newborns (zero to one month) is **70 to 190 bpm** and for infants (one to eleven months) is **80 - 160 bpm.**

It is important to note that there can be variation in these characteristics among individual newborns. If a newborn's characteristics are not close to the norm in any area, please advise the parents to consult with the physician.

Head

Newborns' heads are usually larger in proportion to their bodies than those of older children or adults. If born vaginally, the head will be long and narrow and have possible bruising that will disappear in days or weeks. The baby's head may have:

- Caput: swelling on the top or sides of the head caused by fluid from pressure during labor created from the uterus or vaginal wall. The swellings usually go away after a few days but can last several months after birth.

- "Goose egg": swelling caused by broken blood vessels under the scalp during birth. The swelling may worsen in the first few weeks and take two to three months to disappear.
- Fontanelles: spaces of soft tissue in the skull where the bone is not fully formed, allowing their brains to grow rapidly. There are two noticeable soft spots: the anterior fontanel on top and the posterior fontanel toward the back. These soft spots are crucial for the baby's safe passage through the birth canal; they cushion and protect the head from minor injuries. They also allow the baby's head to absorb falls and soft blows. Although soft, the spots consist of a tough, fibrous membrane, so touching the area is safe. Babies' soft spots come in various sizes at birth and usually enlarge over the first few months. Soft spots will close over within six to eight months.

Hair

Newborns are covered with soft, fine hair called lanugo. This hair is sometimes hard to see and is more common in premature infants. Lanugo most commonly appears on the shoulders and back, but it can also cover the entire infant's body. The hair will fall off about a month after birth.

Babies can be born with varying amounts and colors of hair, while some babies are bald at birth. Most babies will lose the hair they were born with six months after birth, and it is replaced with new hair. Hair color typically changes as they get older.

Hearing

Ears may be soft or folded over and will form a more normal shape within a few days. A dimple or pit in the front of the ear is common, but the baby may need medical attention if there is persistent redness or swelling.

Newborns have fully developed hearing, and babies can orient to the sound of noise and turn toward the side the noise is coming from. During the first month, this works best with the mother's voice. Newborns prefer the mother's voice and the speech patterns/rhythm of the mother's native language since it is familiar to what the baby hears in the womb.

Babies have very sensitive eardrums that loud noises can easily damage. Loud, sudden noises may also startle a baby, so it's advisable to keep noise moderate. It is too loud for the baby if you have to shout over the noise. They prefer rhythmic and soothing sounds like white noise or classical music.

Eyes

Newborns' eyes are usually closed at birth, but they can open them shortly after. Their vision is blurry, and they are most attracted to high-contrast objects. A newborn's eyelids can be swollen for the first several days, and the whites of their eyes can have a red-colored hemorrhage that will go away within six weeks.

An infant's eyes can sometimes appear crossed in the first couple of months; if it persists, inform the baby's doctor.

A newborn's eyes don't make tears until about 6-8 weeks, and their eyes are usually dry. However, watery eyes may occur due to blocked tear ducts, which should open up within a year after birth. You can gently massage and clean the tear duct with a warm washcloth. Inform the baby's doctor if there is a lot of mucus or yellow discharge.

Babies are born with lighter, sometimes grayish eyes, but the color will often change within six months after birth.

Newborns can only see 8 - 12 in. or 20.32 - 30.48 cm., which is about the distance from the mother's breast to her face. They can track objects within the first few weeks, and their eyes will develop normal vision within two to three years.

Newborns prefer light and dark colors versus loud patterns.

Touch

Holding a baby, especially during feedings, is essential to their development. Babies like firm touch or massage because it can make them feel secure.

Swaddling is a technique that provides a sense of security that we will cover more in-depth in a later chapter. Some babies respond well to being "worn" in a sling or carrier.

Taste

Newborns have a preference for the sweet taste of breast milk. They can distinguish between tastes, and variations in the mother's diet can be noticed.

Nose and Smell

The newborn's nose may appear abnormal (flat, unusually large, or pushed in) after birth because of the labor process, but it should appear more normal after a couple of weeks.

Babies have a keen sense of smell that is developed very early in fetal development. They recognize their mother's scent almost immediately, which can comfort them.

It is common for infants to have stuffy noses, and it is important to clean them regularly. It is important to note that infants do not have a *nasomaxillary reflex* at birth and cannot blow their noses. An excellent way to check if they have a stuffy nose is to hold a mirror under each nostril. The nostril is open if mist forms on the mirror. To help with the stuffy nose, you can use saline drops and an aspirator.

Newborns have a unique smell that some people describe as sweet or milky. This smell is thought to result from the amniotic fluid.

Skin

Newborns often have thin, delicate skin covered in **vernix caseosa**, a white, waxy substance that protects the baby's skin from the amniotic fluid. The vernix can appear flaky and dry, especially around the feet, hands, and extremities; this is normal and will peel off in the first couple of weeks. Refrain from using baby lotion and let it peel off naturally since oils and other chemicals can clog the baby's pores.

https://en.wikipedia.org/wiki/Vernix_caseosa

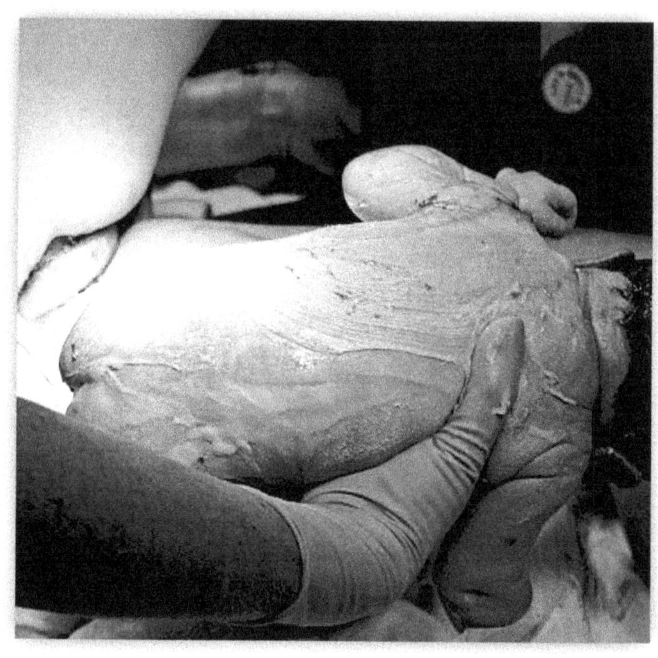

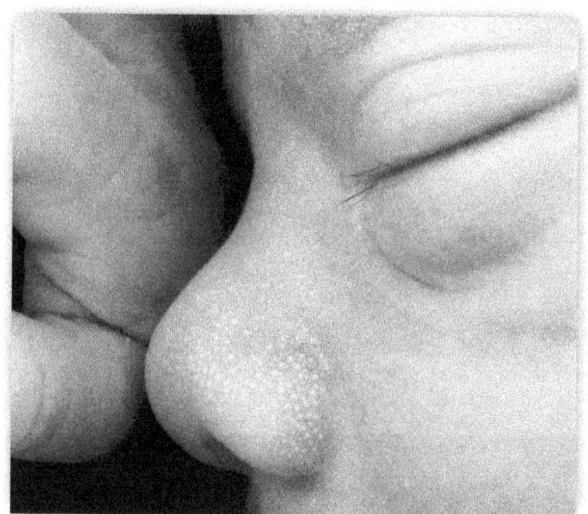

Milia: small white cysts that can appear under the baby's skin, particularly around the nose, eyes, cheeks, and on the roof of their mouth. Milia are very common and benign. Blocked skin pores cause them and typically go away after several weeks when the pores on the baby's skin naturally open. Do not scrub, squeeze, or rub ointments on the milia since it may worsen the cysts.

https://en.m.wikipedia.org/wiki/File:Newborn_Milia_%28Milk_Spots%29.jpg

Erythema toxicum is a very common rash with red blotches with a small white lump in the center. The rash will show up two to five days after birth and will usually go away in one to two weeks. No treatment is needed for the rash.

https://www.momjunction.com/articles/erythema-toxicum-neonatorum-causes-symptoms-treatment_00749638/

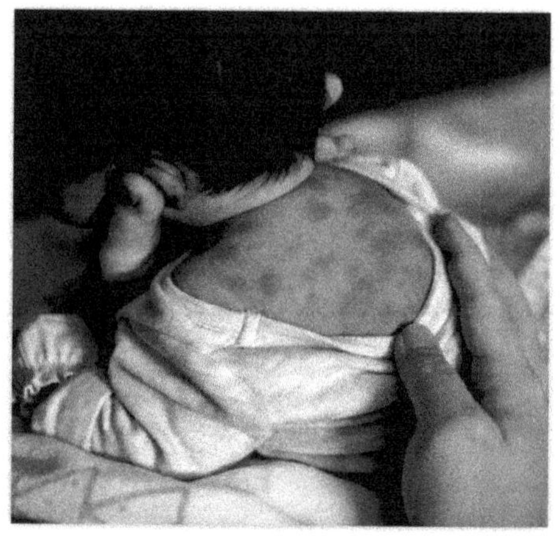

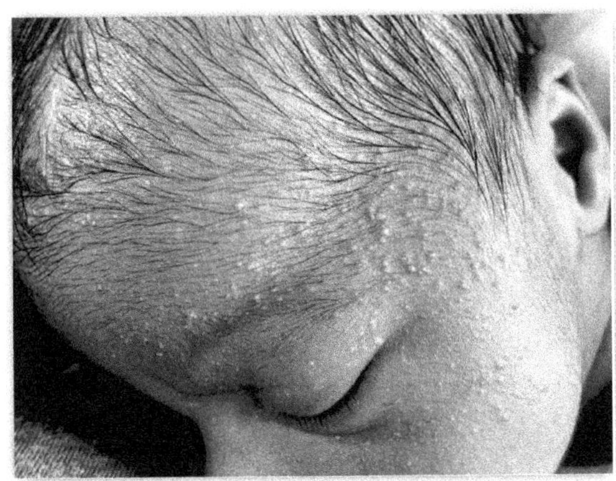

Newborn acne typically begins around two to five weeks after birth and lasts until four to six months. Breastfeeding babies may have these issues a bit longer since hormones from the mother cause the acne. Don't use baby lotion or other creams since they can worsen it. Clean the areas affected with water and soap.

https://www.babycentre.co.uk/l1038755/childhood-rashes-skin-conditions-and-infections-photos

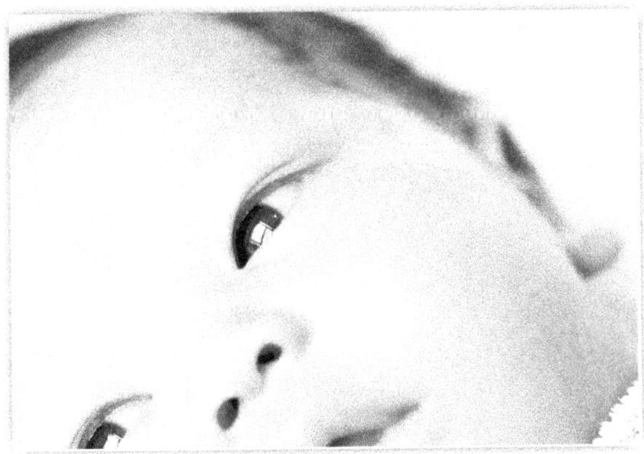

Jaundice is a condition caused by a malfunctioning liver. If an infant has a yellowing of their skin, this could be a sign of jaundice, and the infant should receive medical attention immediately. Jaundice can be challenging to see, especially in infants that have dark skin. An excellent way to check is to gently press the infant's nose or forehead. It could be jaundiced if the skin appears yellow when you lift your finger.

For infants with dark skin, the yellowing of the white parts of the eye may be a more obvious indicator. Read more about the different types of Jaundice in Chapter 18: Baby's Health & Wellness.

https://www.nhs.uk/conditions/jaundice-newborn/symptoms

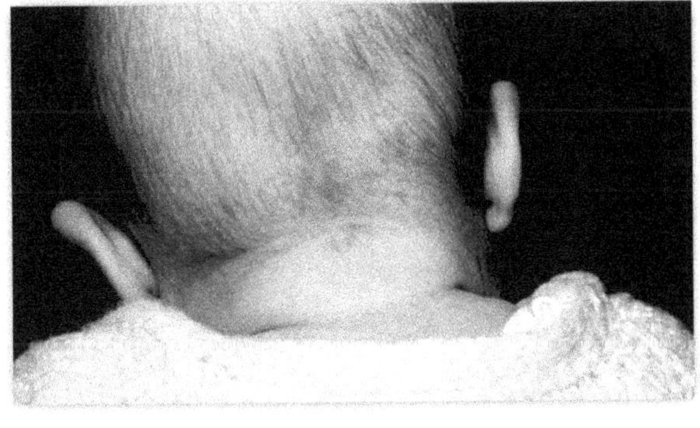

Stork Bites are common birthmarks that are flat, light pink, or burgundy marks on the back of the neck or face. Most of the marks will go away within 18 months. However, some will stay, though they are typically covered by hair.

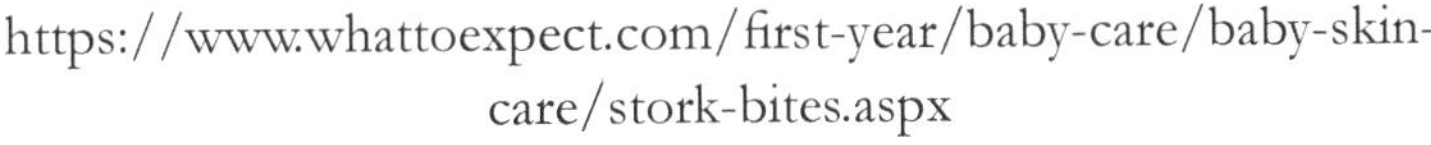

https://www.whattoexpect.com/first-year/baby-care/baby-skin-care/stork-bites.aspx

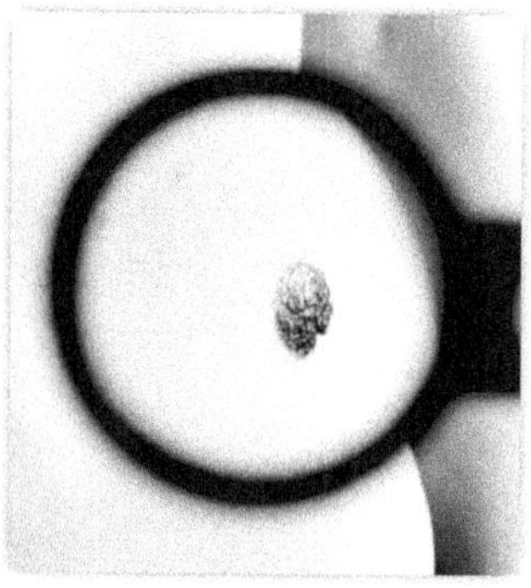

Moles or nevi: Dark brown and black spots that may be on the infant at birth or may be developed over time. Moles are usually harmless and do not need to be removed.

Cafe au lait birthmarks: Flat areas of darkened skin that a These marks are permanent, common, and can occur on any body part.

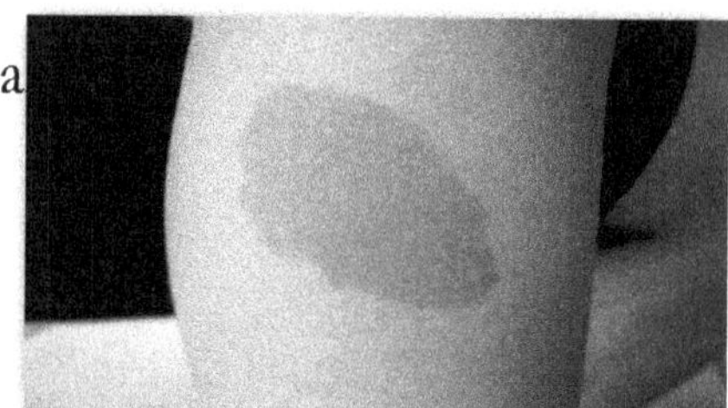

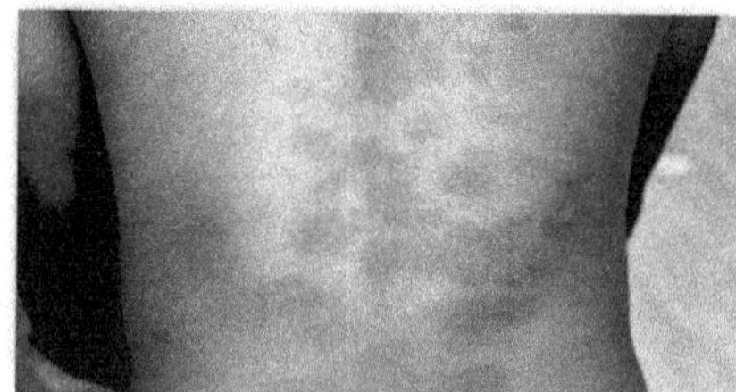

Mongolian blue spots*:* Flat blue-gray birthmarks that appear at or shortly after birth. These marks commonly show up on the shoulders, buttocks, or back. They are harmless and may go away with time.

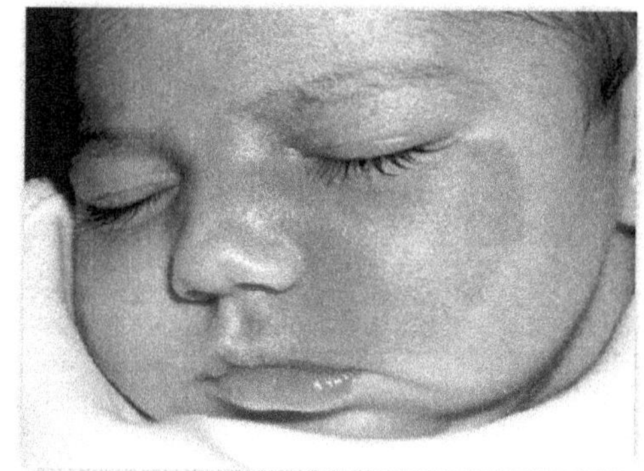

Port Wine Stain*:* Reddish to purplish discoloration caused by dilated capillaries. These can be present at birth and persist throughout life. They can occur anywhere on the body.

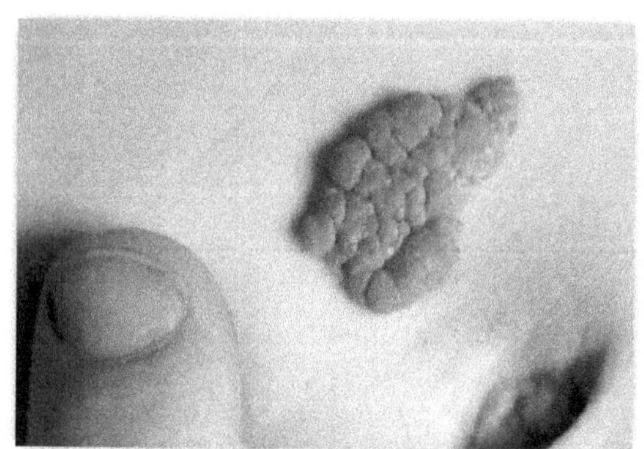

Strawberry Hemangiomas: a clump of blood vessels that form a benign tumor under the skin. The tumor often grows for the first year and then begins to shrink. Most of the hemangiomas fade away by the child's 10th birthday.

Mouth

Being **"tongue-tied"** is an important thing to look for, and it's something doctors and hospitals might miss. A tight frenulum, which you might not see easily in a newborn, can be checked by running a finger under the tongue. A baby with a tight frenulum might have a heart-shaped tongue when crying because the frenulum restricts the upward and forward movement of the tongue. Moms and babies with this issue might experience:

- Painful or damaged nipples
- Slow weight gain
- Long feeds
- Inability to suck for a long time

The following are other mouth issues:

- **Sucking blisters,** found in the center of a baby's upper lip, are from the baby sucking on a thumb, toe, or body part before birth. They're harmless and go away on their own, but it's good to mention them to the doctor to rule out any potential issues.
- **Epithelial pearls** are small, white bumps that form on the gums or hard palate that are roughly the size of a pinhead. These are normal and should clear up within two months.
- **Thrush** is a yeast infection that can result in babies due to a weakened immune system or antibiotic treatments. Thrush produces white patches on the inner cheeks and on the tongue. Inform the infant's doctor or nurse if you think they have thrush.
- **Natal teeth** can be present when a baby is born, but they are uncommon. They are not fully rooted teeth, so they can sometimes cause issues in breastfeeding or be swallowed/ inhaled by the infant. Natal teeth are not the same as neonatal teeth, which erupt in the first month of life.

Check inside the baby's mouth when crying.

Chest

Breast Enlargement: In the first few weeks after birth, newborns may have swollen or enlarged breasts due to hormones being passed onto the infant from the mother. If the infant is breastfeeding, they can have enlarged breasts for a longer duration since hormones are still being passed through the breast milk. The infant may even have spots of milk coming from their breasts, which will go away soon after birth.

Umbilical Cord

Before birth, the umbilical cord provides nutrients and oxygen; after birth, it's clamped and cut. The cord stump should fall off naturally in about two or three weeks. Don't pull or apply anything, but keep it clean and dry. Fold diapers so as not to interfere with the cord.

You may see some yellowish discharge under the dried cord and some bleeding for several days as the cord separates.

Signs Of Infection

- The cord area has an offensive odor.
- Pus-like discharge
- If the area is red, swollen, hot, or tender in an area about an inch to an inch-and-a-half diameter around the cord, these are all signs of infection. Contact the infant's doctor if is the case.

Innies or Outies

The shape of a person's belly button is not determined by how the umbilical cord was cut, but where it was attached.

Female Genitalia

Swollen appearance in the vagina for a few days is normal. Clear, white, pink, or blood-colored discharge may occur and should resolve within one to four weeks.

Male Genitalia

The penis and scrotum make up the external male genitalia. The foreskin is normal and should not be retracted. Erections are common and expected in baby boys. The scrotum may have extra fluid called a hydrocele, which usually goes away in a few months. Undescended testicles may need surgery if not down by age five.

Circumcision

Circumcision refers to the cutting of the foreskin on the male's genitalia. Tenderness and red around the incision should be minimal by the third day. It is expected to see some yellowish coloration on the end of the remaining foreskin or the head of the penis. The scab around the incision usually comes off between the 5th and 10th day.

If a plastic device is used for circumcision, referred to as a Plastibell®, it should fall off within 7-10 days. Make sure to clean the circumcision three times a day with water and apply a healthy amount of Vaseline (avoid touching) to gauze, and place it on the penis before diapering so the circumcision does not stick to the diaper. Use this procedure for four to seven days with every diaper change until there is no more oozing, and the penis looks healthy and pink. Remember always to follow pediatrician recommendations.

Warning Signs

- The normal skin of the penis is red or tender
- Head of the penis is black or blue
- There is dripping blood or a pool of blood in the diaper bigger than a quarter
- The urine stream is weak or comes out in dribbles
- The incision line bleeds more than a few drops
- Any pus is present
- Rectal temperature is over 100.3 or less than 97.5

If any of the above occurs or, if using a Plastibell® ring, it does not fall off within 7-10 days, report to the parents and doctor immediately.

Care Of The Uncircumcised Penis

Many doctors hold the mistaken belief that they must forcefully retract the foreskin of intact, uncircumcised male infants and examine the glans penis. However, this practice is likely to cause pain and harm to the baby as the prepuce is typically too narrow to retract and fused to the underlying glans. Premature retraction can result in the foreskin being torn away from the glans, creating raw surfaces that can lead to adhesions and increase the risk of infection. It is important to inform the physician that no retraction should be performed. Premature retraction of a newborn's foreskin can be considered medical malpractice and may result in legal action.

Umbilical Hernia

When a baby cries or strains, the naval can protrude, and the intestines poke through beneath the skin. This bulge is called an *umbilical hernia.* It may be hardly noticeable, or it may be the size of a golf ball. An opening can occur between the muscles that surround the navel. As the muscles grow, the opening will close, and the hernia will disappear. The hernia is not attractive, but it causes the baby no pain, nor will it harm the baby. Leave it alone. Do not tape it. This could cause more harm than good in the form of infection.

Bowel Movements

A newborn's stool is often yellowish and will have a consistency similar to cottage cheese. However, the color and texture can vary. It is common for a baby to strain when producing stool, even when it is soft. Inform the infant's doctor if the stool is hard or has a clay-like consistency. Also, contact the doctor if the newborn is stooling less than four times daily during the first two weeks after birth.

Toe/Finger Nails

Be cautious when trimming nails, as skin and nails may not have separated. An emery board is recommended for infants to avoid breaking the skin and causing bleeding.

Movements

Newborns have uncoordinated movements and jerky reflexes. They typically have a grasp reflex and a startle reflex. See Chapter 8: Infant Reflexes for a chart of reflexes.

Sleep

Newborns typically sleep for 16-17 hours daily, waking up frequently for feedings.

6.1 How to Interpret the Baby's Signs

Crying is the primary means of communication for newborns. They cry when they are hungry, tired, or uncomfortable. If the baby is not crying or fussing, is alert, aware, and relaxed, it is content and self-soothing. However, suppose the baby is yawning, arching their back, erratically moving their arms or legs, rubbing their eyes, crying, shaking, or won't look at you (caused by over-stimulation). In that case, the baby is likely telling you it is overwhelmed.

Because the baby's cry is its only method of communication, it has no way to express just how urgent their need is. A mild cry might give the impression that the baby has a mild need; an intense cry might reflect an urgent need. But some babies jump past the mild cry into a fierce cry, even though their need is not critical.

6.2 Clues to Look For

Over time, you will learn the baby's signals through their crying. Here are some clues to become familiar with:

- **Breathing rate:** If the breathing is fast or has breaks of two seconds or more, the baby is likely overloaded.
- **Skin color:** If the skin is pale, red, or blotchy, the baby might not feel well. They should have a healthy color.
- **Tone:** What is the tone of their body? Tone is the tension or energy the baby's body reflects when resting. A limp baby is a sign of low tone. As the baby matures, the tone develops, and the baby will begin to curl or tuck the body, starting in the legs and moving up.

- **Posture:** The position of the arms and legs. If stressed, the baby's arms or legs or both might extend. The baby's arms and legs will be curled near the body when relaxed.
- **Movement:** If the baby has stretched arms or splays its toes or fingers, makes fists, protects its face with its arms, has a limp body, or is squirming, it is stressed. If the baby is calm, their movement will be smooth with arms and legs close to the body.
- **Self-Soothing:** If the baby is self-soothing, they are learning to maintain balance. The self-soothing becomes more self-evident as the baby matures. If the baby is doing any of the following, they are starting to use self-soothing:
  - Looking and aware
  - Holding onto or grasping something
  - Bringing hands to face or mouth
  - Hands clasped
  - Sucking behavior
  - Bracing feet and hands together

Chapter 7: The Baby's Mind

The mind of a newborn infant is still a subject of ongoing research and debate among psychologists and neuroscientists. However, some key features of the infant mind are generally accepted:

- Newborn infants have a limited range of sensory and perceptual abilities. They can detect light, sound, touch, and taste, but their vision is blurry, and they cannot focus their eyes on objects or track moving objects until several weeks after birth. They also have a limited ability to differentiate between different sounds and voices.
- Newborn infants have some innate cognitive abilities, such as recognizing human faces and voices. They also have some basic understanding of physical laws, such as the principle of object permanence (the idea that objects continue to exist even when out of sight).
- Newborn infants are highly dependent on their caregivers for survival, and their early experiences and interactions with their caregivers can significantly impact who they become. For example, research has shown that infants who receive responsive and nurturing care in the early months of life tend to develop more secure attachments and better emotional regulation than infants who experience neglect or inconsistent care.

Children's personalities, values, and beliefs are greatly influenced by their parents and other caregivers' actions, attitudes, and behaviors, which can significantly impact their conscious and subconscious development. For example, how parents and other adults communicate with a child has the potential to have an impact on the child's perception of themselves and their environment. For instance, a youngster can create a positive self-image when you use positive affirmations and praise positive behavior.

Children frequently learn by watching and mimicking their parents and other adult caregivers. It is crucial for those who care for children to model virtues like compassion, empathy, and respect. A youngster can also gain a sense of security and self-confidence with the help of regular routines, emotional support, and a secure home environment.

Chapter 8: Infant Reflexes

8.1 Newborn Reflexes

Primitive Reflexes are natural responses we check for in newborns to ensure their neurological and physical development is on track.

8.2 Chart for Normal Reflex Responses

Reflex Name	Stimulus	Response	Time Period (age)	Medical indications & purpose
Palmar Grasp	Stimulate the palm of the infant's hand	Fingers curl inward and clench into a grasp	2-4 months	Test of motor development
Sucking	Touching lips or placing an object in infant's mouth	Tongue moves in the mouth exerting a negative pressure (sucking)	Birth-3 months	Test sucking reflex
Search	Stimulation of area around the mouth	Infant turns head toward the source of stimulation	Birth-11 months	Test search reflex
Moro	Surprise stimulus like a loud noise or allowing the infant's head to drop suddenly backward a short distance (safely)	Sudden extension of arms/legs and spreading of toes and fingers. Limbs then return to flexion position close to the body	Birth-6 months	Used for neurological examination

Reflex Name	Stimulus	Response	Time Period (age)	Medical indications & purpose
Startle	Surprise stimulus like a loud noise or dropping infant's head backward suddenly	Flexion of the limbs close to the body without extension	7-10 months	Neurological examination
Asymmetrical Tonic Neck	Infant placed in supine position with neck turned to the side	The arm extends on the side of the body toward the direction of where the head is turned while the other arm is in a flexed position (lower limbs assume a similar position)	Birth-6 months	Test of Asymmetrical Tonic Neck Reflexes
Symmetrical Tonic Neck	Place infant in a supported sitting position	Extension of head/neck will lead to extension of arms and flexion of legs. If the head/neck are flexed, the infant's arms are flexed with the legs extended	Birth-6 months	Test of Symmetrical Tonic Neck Reflexes
Plantar Grasp	Stroke the sole of the infant's foot	The pressure leads to a contraction of the infant's toes	4-12 months	Neuromuscular system measure
Babinski	Stroke the sole of the infant's foot	The pressure leads to an extension of the infant's toes	Birth-3 months	Neuromuscular system measure
Palmar Mental reflex	Scratching base of the infant's palm	The scratching causes a contraction of the chin muscles, lifting the infant's chin upward	Birth-2 months	Test hand-mouth reflexes
Palmar Mandibular	Apply pressure to the palms of both hands	The responses usually include mouth opening, closing of the eyes, and moving the head forward	Birth-3 months	Test hand-mouth reflexes

Reflex Name	Stimulus	Response	Time Period (age)	Medical indications & purpose
Stepping	The infant is held upright with the body weight placed forward on a flat surface	Infant will perform a walking movement with their legs	Birth-4 months	Test walking reflexes
Crawling	Infant placed in a prone position and pressure is applied to the sole of one foot	Reflexive crawling using the upper and lower limbs	Birth-3 months	Test for reflexive crawling
Swimming	Place infant in prone position in water	Flexor swimming movements of arms and legs	Birth-12 months	Test for neck and body-righting reflexes
Head and body (neck/ body) righting	Infant placed in supine position with head turned to one side	Infant's body moves reflexively in the same direction of the head	Birth-12 months	Test for neck and body-righting reflexes
Parachuting	Enactment of sudden displacing force or loss of balance	Protective movements of the infant's limbs in the direction of the displacing force	4-12 months	Tests for parachute reflexes
Labyrinthine	Infant is held in an upright position and is tilted to the side, forward, or backward	Infant will move in the opposite direction to the direction it is displaced to maintain the upright position of the head	2-6 months	Test for the Labyrinth reflex

Reflex Name	Stimulus	Response	Time Period (age)	Medical indications & purpose
Pull-up	Infant is in upright sitting position and is held up by one or both hands and is tipped backward or forward	Infant flexes its arms to remain in the upright sitting position	3-12 months	Test for pull-up reflex
Steriotypies	Natural process before voluntary movement develops	Rhythmic movements performed continusously for their own sakes	Birth-12 months	Rhythmic movements increase just before infant gains voluntary control of that system

8.3 Reflexes at 3-4 Months

At three to four months of age, the automatic reflexes in babies are going away or weakening. Although it's not perfect, they're starting to control their hands and feet more. The baby might begin using both hands together for certain things. Even though they can't fully grab items yet, they can try to bring objects closer by swiping at them.

When lying on their tummy, babies can lift their upper body, shoulders, and head using their arms. Their neck muscles are strengthening, allowing them to sit with some support and hold their head up. Also, their eyes are getting better at following things.

Chapter 9: Milestones Through the First Year of Life

Babies will quickly grow and develop in their first year of life. Most babies will double their weight within the first six months and triple it by their first year. Developmental milestones can be helpful to understand better where a child is in their development compared to the "average" child. However, it is essential to note that every baby is unique and will develop at their own pace. Most babies will reach certain milestones around the same ages, but it is perfectly normal for healthy babies to fall behind in some areas and be ahead in others. Milestones should be seen as guidelines to aid in evaluating the baby's development, but understand that they are imperfect measurements.

Also, note that a premature baby will compare to the milestones differently. When looking at the milestones for premature babies, base it on their expected due date and not their actual birthday. For example, if the baby is born one month premature, you should expect them to achieve milestones about a month later than the guidelines predict.

9.1 One-Month Milestones

- Recognition of sounds, especially the parents' voices
- Good hearing
- Hands are in tight fists
- Able to bring hands near the face
- Jerking arm movements
- Ability to move head side to side when lying on their stomach
- Preference/recognition of human faces compared to other shapes
- Preference for high-contrast patterns and black-and-white
- Ability to focus on objects within an 8- to 12-inch distance

9.2 Three-Month Milestones

- Cooing and making soft sounds
- Begin to babble and imitate sounds
- More directed cries (hunger, pain, anger, boredom)
- Enjoys playing with other people and may cry when play stops
- Smiling, especially when parents speak
- Opening and shutting hands
- Grasping objects
- Coordination between hands and eyes begin
- Ability to follow moving objects with eyes
- Recognition of faces and familiar objects at a farther distance
- Support of the upper body with arms and able to raise chest while laying on stomach
- Can stretch legs out and kick
- Can push down on legs when feet are on a firm surface

9.3 Six-Month Milestones

- Explores objects with mouth and hands
- Reaches for objects with hands
- Transfers objects between hands
- Development of mature vision
- Likes to play peek-a-boo
- Enjoys looking at mirror images
- Can distinguish emotions by tone of voice
- Can recognize their name
- Consonant babble chains (ba-ba-ba)
- Expresses joy or distress with their voice
- Rolls over from stomach to back and back to stomach
- Can support their weight on their legs when they are held upright
- Ability to sit up

9.4 One-Year Milestones

- Explores objects in more complex ways (throwing, dropping, shaking)
- Can use simple objects correctly (drinking from a cup)
- Can find hidden objects
- Looks at correct image when it is named
- Simple gesturing like waving or shaking the head
- Simple words like "mama," "dada," and "uh-oh"
- Imitates words
- Responds to simple verbal requests
- Can crawl
- Can sit without assistance
- Can stand by pulling themselves up
- Walks while being supported
- Sometimes takes a few steps without support
- Uses thumb and forefinger (pincer grasp)

Chapter 10: Premature Infants

Babies born from 37 to 42 weeks are considered "full-term." All infants born before 37 weeks and weighing less than 3 lbs. 8 oz. are called "premature." Premature births occur in roughly one in ten babies born in the U.S., and Newborn Care Specialists must be aware of some of the challenges that may accompany premature infants.

Generally, babies can sustain life after 25 weeks of gestation, but being born prematurely can often lead to many health complications, and many premature infants need to spend days, weeks, or even months in the newborn intensive care unit (NICU).

After 25 weeks of pregnancy, the main focuses for the baby are maintaining body temperature, breathing on their own, and gaining weight. Sometimes, they might get steroids before birth to help their lungs develop. Other things, like nails growing and eyebrows forming, also happen during this stage of development.

Terms used to describe premature infants:

Late preterm: infant born between 34-36 weeks of gestation

Moderate preterm: infant born between 32-34 weeks of gestation

Very preterm: infant born between 26-32 weeks of gestation

Extremely preterm: infant born at or before 25 weeks of gestation

Micro preemies: infant who weighs less than 1lb. 12oz. and are generally born before 25 weeks of gestation.

Premature babies are born with minimal fat and thin skin. Their organs are formed but might not work well because they are not mature enough. Babies born between 30 and 34 weeks typically weigh between 2 lbs. 3oz. - 5 lbs. 8oz. Any baby born between 34-37 weeks could face some of the same difficulties as a very premature infant.

10.1 Common Complications for Premature Infants

- Neurological developmental issues and delays
- Physical disabilities
- Increased risks of infections or neonatal sepsis
- Abnormal development in the brain, lungs, heart, or other organs
- Intraventricular hemorrhage (IVH): bleeding in fluid-filled spaces in the brain
- Anemia: issues with producing healthy red blood cells
- Newborn jaundice: yellowish discoloration of the skin due to immature liver function
- Necrotizing enterocolitis (NEC): damage in the newborn's intestines
- Retinopathy of prematurity (ROP): eye disease that occurs when the retinas don't fully develop
- Incomplete/incompetent feeding reflexes

10.2 Difficulties Premature Infants May Experience

- Reaching/maintaining a healthy body weight
- Breathing issues, including apnea, especially during sleep
- Feeding issues
- Body temperature regulation
- Other challenges based on specific health complications

10.3 Requirements for Release from the Hospital

An infant will only be discharged when the following happens:

- Their body temperature is maintained
- They are steadily gaining weight
- They feed from a bottle, not a feeding tube
- They breathe on their own
- They reach a healthy body weight

Most preemies will be able to accomplish the list above 2-3 weeks before their original due date. What will change is if they have extenuating circumstances like having malformations, requiring oxygen, spending weeks on a breathing machine, or have had surgery; in those cases, they would need to stay in the hospital beyond the due date.

10.4 Caring for a Premature Infant

Premature infants can quickly become overstimulated, so it is vital to identify when the baby is distressed and know how to calm it.

If you see the baby getting upset, like a change in color or restlessness, stop and gently place your open hand on the baby's back or stomach. If the baby seems okay, you can softly stroke the infant. Speak quietly using gentle tones because premature infants are sensitive to noise and lights; keep these to a minimum. If the distress continues, stop and try again later.

If the nursery has bright colors or toys, you might need to make the room darker. Preemies can be too sensitive to handle such things. Moving the baby to a less colorful area or using a white sheet around the crib can help reduce stimulation.

Touch might be too much for a preemie. Even though you may want to hold the tiny baby, it could be overwhelming for them. Let them sleep in a dark, quiet space if that's the case.

10.5 Tips for Sleep and Holding

- Premature infants should be swaddled most of the time since this makes them feel safe and reminds them of being in the womb. The preemie swaddle technique is the best (you will receive instructions for this technique in Chapter 13: Swaddling).
- Body carriers such as slings may be very effective in consoling the infant. However, it is important to occasionally put them down when they are awake to help them learn self-soothing techniques.
- If you are rocking the infant, limit the noise and shield their eyes from light to prevent overstimulation. Always pay attention to signals of distress and, if necessary, decrease the intensity of the rocking to a slower pace. If they are still signaling distress, the baby may need to rest in a darkened and quiet space.
- Refrain from fast movements and loud noises. Make sure to handle the infant slowly, methodically, and gently.
- To provide additional comfort while sleeping, place the baby's hands near their face/ mouth or offer them a pacifier to suckle.

10.6 Tips for Feeding

- Limit other stimuli while the baby is feeding since eating can be a lot of work for them. This can be done by feeding in a quiet, darkened room.
- If the infant falls asleep while feeding, wake the infant to conclude the feeding by gently rubbing their head or feet, unswaddling them, or burping them.

- Premature infants may need to feed more often at shorter intervals.

10.7 Adjusted Age Explained

Adjusted age is the developmental age based on the due date. If a baby was due on Jan 14th and was born on Jan 1st, on Jan 31st, the actual age would be four weeks old, but the baby's adjusted age would only be two weeks old. Some babies catch up to their actual age fast, and some are slower.

Homework for Section 2

- How to care for an umbilical cord?
- What is circumcision? How do you care for it during a bath or a diaper change?
- What is self-soothing? Give examples.
- What is adjusted age in preemies?

Section 3: Practical and Effective Infant Care

Chapter 11: Nursery Necessities and Safety Tips

Here are some nursery necessities and suggestions to help you get started. The following are divided into Necessities and Helpful Additions.

11.1 Necessities

- Clothing: A baby can go through many outfits from the day of arrival through toddlerhood. Have a quarter of the baby clothes be in the 0-3 month size and the rest in the 3-6 month size. If it is a preemie baby, they will only wear gowns as they will not be going out. Increase the amounts depending on how many multiples.
- Bottles: Six BPA-free four-ounce bottles. If there are multiples, buy bottles with different colored nipple rings and assign a color to each baby.
- Slow-flow Nipples: Review nipple size often. If the flow is too slow the baby has to work too hard, potentially causing slow weight gain. As the baby gets older you can use faster-flowing nipples.
- Diapers and wipes: Stock the diaper changing area with plenty of diapers and wipes for the night. You'll be surprised how quickly you go through them! Encourage the parents to choose diapers and wipes without chemicals.
- Diaper pail: A diaper pail can help keep odors under control and make diaper changes more convenient. Use a liner to make clean-up easier. A flip-top or locking lid can help contain odors. You can add baking soda to the bottom to help absorb odors. Be sure to empty at the end of every shift.
- Crib: A safe and comfortable place for the baby to sleep is essential. Ensure the crib meets safety standards.
- Crib sheets: Have at least three on hand, as one is invariably in the washer, and having three provides a backup. Avoiding bright patterns is recommended, as some babies are

easily overstimulated and have trouble sleeping. Also, avoid sheets that feel like a t-shirt (jersey-type) or anything inexpensive, as these usually don't fit the crib well, and babies tend to pull on them.

- Crib Sheet Savers: Cloth pads that tie onto the crib to save you from having to change the crib sheets. It is suggested to have at least three for the same reason as having three crib sheets.
- Mattress: We recommend that the parent invest in a good quality mattress that fits snugly in the crib. Ensure the mattress is firm and supports the baby's developing spine.
- Rocking chair or glider: A comfortable place to sit while feeding, rocking, or soothing the baby can be a lifesaver.
- Baby monitor: A baby monitor allows you to monitor the baby when you're in another room.
- Swaddle blankets: Swaddling can help soothe the baby and promote better sleep (more about swaddling in Chapter 13). We recommend blankets made from soft, breathable material. Have at least four swaddling blankets. These are different than receiving blankets, which are not useful for swaddling.
- Burp cloths: Whether the baby is being bottle-fed or breastfed, you will need plenty of burp cloths to clean up any messes. Cloth diapers are the best because they can easily be cleaned and replaced.
- Onesies and sleepers: The baby will spend most of their time in these cozy, one-piece outfits. We recommend onesies and sleepers made from natural, soft, breathable material. You can request sleepers that snap or zip all the way to the feet for ease of getting the baby into it.
- Hand soap: Place a pump bottle at every sink.
- Diaper rash cream: Essential to prevent a sore bottom. We recommend organic products as some babies are very sensitive.
- Gauze and salve for circumcision: 4x4 gauze pads and a tub of Vaseline.
- Formula: There are many choices but we recommend organic goat or cow's milk, if possible. As an NCS, you can make recommendations, but this choice is up to the parents and pediatrician.
- Bibs for feeding: Bibs help cut down on laundry. We recommend bibs that velcro or snap closed instead of ties, which can be dangerous. A baby sleeping in a bib is not recommended; bibs are for feeding and burping only.

- Infant car seat with head supporter.
- Diaper bag with portable changing pad.
- Nasal aspirator: An aspirator can be a life-saver during the first few weeks of a baby's life. Get a small bulb syringe-type that disassembles for easier cleaning.
- Saline drops: Very important for comfortable nasal aspiration.
- Thermometers: Rectal is the most accurate. Ear thermometers are only recommended for babies three months or older. Forehead thermometers are not recommended.
- Vaseline or other non-chemical ointment: To use with thermometers or for circumcision bandages.
- Night light: Avoid using bright lights at night. We suggest using a reading light with an attached clamp that can be mounted on the changing table, etc.

11.2 Helpful Additions

- Newborn gowns: Gowns are easier than snaps at night when a baby is crying on the changing table. Even during the day, gowns are more efficient; babies need about 12 diaper changes per day for the first few weeks.
- Bottle sterilizer and drying rack
- Bottle/nipple brush
- Breast pump and breast milk storage bags if breastfeeding
- Changing table with drawers: A changing table or dresser with a changing pad on top can make diaper changes easier and more organized.
- Changing table pads: These small, waterproof pads will help when there is a messy change; you only have to wash the pad versus the entire table cover.
- Baby bathtub: A small baby bathtub can make bath time easier and safer for the little one.
- Sound machine: A white noise sound machine can help soothe the baby to sleep and drown out any outside noise. The deeper the sound, the more relaxing; higher pitches are more stimulating. Avoid waves, birds, or heartbeats, and use the white or brown noise options.
- Baby emery board for carefully filing a baby's fingernails. Nail clippers or scissors can cause injury to the baby.
- Liquid baby soap: We recommend organic products only.

- Baby hairbrush
- Small space heater for cold climates
- Colic remedies
- Pacifiers: Helps with fussy periods and when the baby needs non-food sucking. Use a one-piece design.
- Bouncy seat: Great for keeping the baby occupied during awake time.
- Swing: This can be helpful with a fussy baby for short periods of time.
- Electric clock with light-up display: Essential for knowing when to feed.
- Stroller: We recommend a stroller that is easy to fold, portable, and maneuvers well. If it has a removable car seat, it's even better.

For Multiples

- A twin boppy or something similar
- A prop to hold a second bottle (use multiple towels or rags or rice socks)

11.3 Crib Safety Considerations

The **American Academy of Pediatrics (AAP)** recommends that all infants sleep on their backs with nothing in the crib unless otherwise advised by your pediatrician or if the baby has reflux. We recommend using rice socks or an infant positioner.

- **Crib slats:** The slats should be no more than 2-3/8 inches apart. All new cribs must meet this standard, but older cribs may not. Avoid using any crib that does not meet the **2024** standard.
- **Bumpers and no pillows:** We recommend mesh bumper pads and no pillows in the crib for safety.
- **Crib toys:** We don't recommend having any toys in the crib. Do not tie or suspend toys from the crib bars unless specifically made to connect to the side (they usually have plastic attachments).
- **Mobiles**: Mobiles are a great source of stimulation for the baby, providing entertainment. However, it can also be a distraction for sleeping. Have one with a swivel arm to move it out of the range of vision when needed. If the parent chooses to use a mobile, make sure it does not hang low enough to entangle the baby. Once the baby can sit up, it's time to take them down.

- **Baby's mattress:** We recommend a mattress that fits snugly in the crib. You should be able to get no more than two fingers between the mattress and crib slats. Many mattresses off-gas; buying a non-toxic mattress is important. If the family cannot afford a non-toxic mattress, a polyethylene mattress cover is recommended to block off-gassing; the cover does not off-gas itself. A good source of information about mattresses is HealthyChild.com.
- **Bedding:** Snug, breathable, natural-cloth fitted mattress sheets are recommended. No loose bedding in the crib.
- **Tooth-resistant rails:** Some railings are covered by special plastic to prevent teething babies from gnawing on the paint or wood.
- **Adjustable mattress height:** Many cribs have adjustable heights so you can lower the mattress as the baby gets taller, making it more difficult for them to climb out. Always be aware of the mattress height and when it needs to be changed.

11.4 Bassinet Safety

Many parents choose to have a bassinet because they can keep it near their bed, and it's easy to move from one room to another. The AAP approves bassinets as a safe sleep space for the newborn.

- Ensure the bassinet is stable and doesn't pose a potential tipping hazard.
- Only use a bassinet for the first three to four months.
- Babies weighing over 20 pounds should not be placed in a bassinet.
- Ensure there is no loose bedding.

11.5 Changing-Table Safety

Although a changing table makes it easier to dress and diaper the baby, falls from such a high surface can be serious. The top of the changing table should be concave so the middle is slightly lower than the edges to hold a baby in place more naturally.

Buckle the safety strap, but also always keep a hand on the baby. **Never leave a child unattended on a changing table, even for a moment**—even if they are strapped.

Keep diapering supplies within your reach but out of the child's so that you don't have to leave the baby's side while they are on the changing table.

11.6 Infant Seats/Bouncies and Swing Safety

- Always use the safety straps that come with the seat. There should be a crotch and waist strap.
- Make sure the seat is sturdy and stable with a wide bottom.
- If you set it on the table or counter, be sure it's not too close to the edge.
- Never leave a baby unattended, even when they are strapped in the seat.
- Do not set the seat on a bed, couch, or surface where it can tip over or slide off.

11.7 Bedroom Safety

- Keep nightlights away from drapes or bedding where they could start a fire. Use only cool nightlights that do not get hot.
- It's best to have smoke alarms and carbon dioxide detectors in every bedroom.
- Ensure the crib or bouncy seats are not close to window blinds, drapes, or cords to prevent the baby from getting caught in cords.
- Do not place the crib under a vent where cold or hot air may come out.
- Do not hang heavy pictures over the crib.
- Look for lights that may affect baby's sleep. (Lights on monitors, chargers, etc.).
- Room should be cool and dark (68-72 degrees is recommended). Cover any lights that may affect baby's sleep.

Chapter 12: Caring for a Newborn's Basic Needs

This chapter covers the basic tasks you will be performing daily, including diapering and bathing.

12.1 Diapering

Diapering a newborn can seem daunting initially, but it will become second nature with some practice. Here are the steps to follow.

- Gather your supplies: You will need clean diapers, wipes, diaper rash cream (if needed), and a changing pad or blanket.
- Prepare the changing area: Lay the baby on the changing pad or blanket, making sure it's a clean, flat surface. If you're using a changing table, secure the safety strap.
- Wash Hands
- Place the new diaper under the infant before you take the old diaper off.
- With a boy, have an extra piece of cloth or diaper ready to lie across his penis, or you may receive a shower. (Urine is 100% sterile as it comes out of the body. The bacterium happens after it is exposed to air.)
- Remove the dirty diaper: Unfasten the tabs on the dirty diaper and gently lift the baby's legs by the ankles, supporting their bottom with one hand. Use the front of the diaper to wipe away any poop or pee, then fold the dirty diaper in half and set it aside.
- Clean the baby: Using a washcloth or baby wipes, gently wipe the baby clean from the front to the back. Never wipe from the back to the front, as this can cause urinary tract infections. Use a clean wipe for each swipe, and continue until the baby is clean and dry. You may want to lift the baby's legs to get a better reach. Don't forget the little creases in the thighs and buttocks. Pat dry.
- Apply diaper cream (if needed): If the baby has a diaper rash, apply a thin layer of diaper cream to the affected area after properly washing it (see section below on diaper rash).

- Pull the front of the new diaper that is currently under the baby up between their legs and fasten the tabs on each side.
- Dispose of the dirty diaper: Roll up the dirty diaper and fasten the tabs together. Place it in a diaper pail or plastic bag for disposal.
- Wash Hands: Use a wipe or clean washcloth.
- Dress the baby: Put on a fresh outfit if needed, and you are done!

Additional Tips

- If you find marks around the baby's legs or waist, the diaper is too tight.
- If a rash develops over the entire area where the diaper touches the baby, the baby may be allergic to the diaper or the detergent the diapers are washed in. Try different bleach-free brands for sensitive skin.
- When diapering a boy, place the penis in a downward position before fastening the diaper. This will prevent leaks.
- Fold the plastic down to prevent leaks from coming over the top of the diaper.
- Until the umbilical cord is healed and drops off, diaper the baby with the diaper folded to stay under the cord. The diaper is never to rub or cover the umbilical cord as this can lead to infection.

Disposable Diapers

Most mothers now are choosing to use disposable diapers. They save the hassle of manually washing cloth diapers. If a baby has an allergic reaction to the disposable diaper, you may suggest they try an organic or more natural, bleach-free brand of diapers.

Washing Cloth Diapers

If you have a mom who insists on using cloth diapers, she will tell you how she wants them cared for. DiaperPin.com has some good washing instructions for cloth diapers, and we have included them below:

- Pre-Wash: Place all cloth diapers in the washer and run a pre-wash in cold water. This will remove most of the loose particles from the cloth diapers.
- Overnight Soak: Refill the washer with cold water and ½-cup of baking soda. Baking soda is a base and neutralizes the urine in cloth diapers; this is also very effective in whitening and removing the smell from cloth diapers. Let it agitate for a minute or two, then turn off the machine and let the cloth diapers soak for several hours or overnight. Drain the water (run another pre-wash).

- Hot Wash: Run the wash with hot water, detergent, and ½-cup baking soda. Since a baby has sensitive skin, use a hypoallergenic detergent.
- Double Rinse: Add about ½-cup vinegar during the first rinse. If you have a washer with a fabric softener compartment, pour the vinegar there when starting the hot wash. For the second rinse, use cold water.
- No Soak Method: If you prefer not to soak your diapers, run a regular wash cycle.

Diaper Rash

The following chart lists types of diaper rashes and possible solutions:

Name of Rash	Appearance of Rash	Solution to Rash
Allergic Reaction	Red ring around the anus	Check the diet: for formula, change brands; if breastfeeding, what is mom eating?
Contact Dermatitis	Appears as flat, red, irritated skin around thighs, waist, or anywhere diaper is rubbing. Does not typically appear in the folds of the skin. Will blister or peel and slough off when severe.	Often caused by chemicals in the diaper. Change brands; look for bleach-free at a health food store.
Impetigo	Raised, coin-sized patches or blisters oozing from a honey-colored crust that appear around the buttocks and groin.	This is a strep infection. See doctor as soon as possible to get an antibiotic cream prescription.
Intertrigo	Heat and moisture retention that is irritated by urine. Red and burn-like in appearance that is found in the folds of the skin.	Make sure baby is cool and dry and check diapers frequently.
Seborrhea Dermatitis	Red, raised, rough, and oily-looking over the diaper area.	Cortisone cream (1/2 – 1%). Use very little to prevent damage to the skin and only until rash is gone. NEVER use as a preventative.

Yeast Rash (Thrush)	Tiny red or pink, raised rash that might appear on top of another rash. If no methods work to remove the rash, suspect yeast. Check inside the mouth for white patches. The source can be from mom during delivery, a caregiver, or too much yeast in their system. Yeast spreads, so wash hands after touching any affected area.	Lotrimin Cream Or, if you prefer natural: ➤ Baking soda wash (1 tsp baking soda dissolved in 1 cup of water). Pat on baby's bum and swab inside baby's mouth. ➤ Swab baby's mouth and mom's breast with plain yogurt after feeding. ➤ If bottle-fed, boil all nipples and bottles each use for two weeks after symptoms disappear. ➤ Wash all bedding in hot water, using white vinegar in final rinse.

If the baby is getting the rash from commercial wipes, use inexpensive washcloths, paper towels cut in half, or a cut up towel (flannel or other cotton fabric) with the edges finished.

Consult the doctor if:

- Pimples and small ulcers form
- The baby loses weight or isn't eating as well as usual
- Large bumps or nodules appear
- The rash spreads
- The rash occurs in the first six weeks of life

12.2 Bathing

Bathing a newborn can be a delicate task, and it's important to take extra care to keep the baby safe and comfortable during the process. Here are some general steps you can follow:

1. **Gather your supplies:** You will need a clean, warm towel, mild baby soap, a washcloth or sponge, a clean diaper, and a change of clothes.

2. **Fill the tub or sink with warm water:** The water should be about two to three inches deep. Be sure it is very warm while preparing the bath; it will cool down fast, so watch the temperature. Babies generally like it warm rather than cool. It must be between 98.6° - 99.6° F. for optimal comfort (comfortably warm to your inner wrist or elbow).
3. **Undress the baby:** Make sure the room is warm to prevent the baby from getting cold.
4. **Support the baby:** Hold the baby gently but securely, using one hand to support their head and neck.
5. **Wet the baby:** Use a washcloth or sponge to wet the baby's body, being careful to avoid getting water in their eyes, nose, or mouth.
6. **Wash the baby:** Use a small amount of mild baby soap to wash the baby's body, starting with their face and working your way down to their toes. Pay extra attention to creases and folds where dirt and sweat can accumulate.
7. **Rinse the baby:** Use a washcloth or cup to rinse the baby thoroughly, again being careful to avoid getting water in their face.
8. **Dry the baby:** Use a clean, soft towel to gently pat the baby dry, paying extra attention to the creases and folds. Don't rub the baby's skin too hard, which can irritate it.
9. **Follow with a baby massage:** Use coconut oil or an organic baby lotion.
10. **Dress the baby:** Once the baby is dry, put on a clean diaper and dress them in clean clothes.

Always keep a hand on the baby during the bath and never leave them unattended in the water, even for a moment. **DO NOT LEAVE THE ROOM. DO NOT TALK OR TEXT ON YOUR CELL PHONE**. You need to give the situation your undivided attention.

As the baby gets older, they will get more active in the bath, and you may be a bit wet from all the splashing. As the baby learns to sit up, there is a tub chair you can sit them in, and they will love this.

We recommend that multiples are bathed separately. However, some sources recommend bathing twins by placing them head to head in the bath to save time. If you choose to do this, please do not take your eyes off the babies. When it is time to take them out, you will take out one, drying and diapering that baby by the bath, keeping your eye on the other baby. As they get older, it will be easier, as you can sit them both up.

When the baby gets too big for the sink or baby tub, you can transition into the adult tub but start with only a couple of inches of water. Lay a mat on the bottom of the tub and place the baby in the water and on its back. Keep the baby's nose out of the water, but it is fine if water gets in the ears. Make sure not to split your attention or leave the room while the baby is in the adult bath. It can help to have a heater in the bathroom to keep the bathroom nice and warm.

You can allow the baby as much time in the tub as they want. It will wear them out and is great to do before their nap.

It is important to note that full baths should not be given until the umbilical cord has fully detached and healed. Similarly, if the infant has a circumcision, wait until it is healed before starting full baths. In the meantime, give the baby a sponge bath.

Sponge Bath

- Fill the sink with warm water and make sure to have a towel, soap, and a washcloth ready.
- Remove the infant's clothing and cover them in a thin blanket for warmth. As you wash different areas of the infant, it is important to unwrap the blanket as you bathe the area and re-cover it when you are done to keep the baby warm and comfortable.
- Use a non-chemical soap that will not irritate the infant's skin, and lather the soap onto the washcloth.
- Gently rub the washcloth on the infant's skin and rinse each area with another clean washcloth when you are done. Make sure to clean the area that is normally covered by the diaper especially well and roll the baby over to wash their back.
- It is normal for infants to cry during a sponge bath. Just make sure to wash the infant gently and keep them at a warm temperature.

12.3 Clothing Guidelines

The American Academy of Pediatrics recommends the ideal temperature for a baby's comfort to be between 68°and 72° F. These clothing rules are from experience only, and there is no scientific evidence that this is correct.

Over 80° - Diaper and 100% thin cotton swaddling blanket

75-80° - Diaper, t-shirt, and swaddling blanket

70-75° - Diaper, gown, swaddling blanket

Below 70° - Diaper, gown, and double swaddle

Chapter 13: Swaddling

Swaddling is a traditional practice of wrapping a newborn baby snugly in a blanket or cloth to provide a sense of security and comfort. This practice has been used for centuries in various cultures and is believed to help soothe fussy babies, prevent startle reflexes, provide protection from the elements, and promote better sleep. Swaddling helps the infant transition from womb to life, and it is an important tool for allowing the parents and baby time to rest.

Swaddling is typically done by wrapping the baby in a blanket or cloth, snugly but not too tight, with the arms tucked in and the legs straight. It is vital to ensure that the baby's hips can move freely and that the swaddle is not too tight around the chest or neck.

Swaddling from zero to three months is very important since newborns don't have much control over their limbs and don't know when they are thrashing their arms around. Swaddling keeps their arms tucked, preventing an infant from scratching their face or startling themselves awake by moving their limbs. It also prepares the baby to sleep on their side since their tucked-in limbs make it less likely that the baby will turn over into a prone position.

Between three and four months, you can start using a transition swaddle like Merlin's Magic Sleepsuit or Dreamland Swaddle, which helps the baby get used to sleeping without a swaddle. After four months, the baby should be sleeping on their own without any swaddling.

13.1 When to Swaddle

- If the infant is overstimulated or is crying uncontrollably, swaddling can help the baby settle down.
- Swaddle the baby if they are flailing their arms or scratching their face. Swaddling can calm the baby's movement and prevent them from hurting or startling themselves.
- Swaddle infants at night and for naps in the first three months. If you swaddle infants in a consistent pattern, it will be easier for the baby to transition to sleep schedules without swaddling.
- Swaddle if the baby is difficult to feed; the swaddle controls movement and calms them.

- You can stop swaddling if the baby is moving around the crib, if the baby can roll over, or any time after four months

13.2 How to Swaddle

Baby Burrito Wrap

1. Put your baby in the middle of the blanket with the neck even with the top of the center of the blanket.
2. Take the first corner, bring it under the baby's chin, forming a 'v,' and wrap it under the baby's body, holding one or both arms down by the sides.
3. Take the other side, wrap it around the baby, forming another 'v,' pull it tightly, and wrap it around.
4. Fan out the bottom of the blanket, bring it up to the right under the baby's chin, and wrap each wing tightly around it.

Dr. Karp's Swaddle

1. Lay the blanket wrong-side-up on a flat surface. Fold the top corner down to the center of the blanket. Place the baby so the neck is on the folded edge.
2. Hold the baby's right arm straight at the baby's side. Pull the blanket tightly down and across the baby's body. Tuck it under the baby's left buttock and lower back, keeping it tight. The baby's right arm should not move.
3. Straighten the baby's left arm against the side, and bring the bottom corner up and over the baby's left shoulder. Hold the left arm against the body and tuck the blanket under it.
4. Fold the top of the blanket down a little, making a V-neck shape. Hold it in place and pull the remaining corner tightly to the right, wrapping it across the baby's body like a wide belt. Tuck the end into the front of the belt.
5. Make sure it's tight across the chest/arms. The baby should feel secure.

Remember, it's okay if the baby doesn't like it initially, but a snug swaddle helps them feel secure. Allow the hips to move freely; tightness is most important across the chest/arms.

Tips for Swaddling Safely

- Leave the legs completely out of the swaddle. Do not straighten the baby's legs or bind them together with the swaddle. The legs should be allowed to curl and straighten at will.
- Always lay the swaddled baby on their back.

- Ensure that the swaddle is not too tight or too loose. Dr. Karp suggests "as tight as the waistband on the mother's pants just before the baby is born." If too loose, you run the risk of loose blankets in the crib, making it easier to smother the baby.
- Avoid crossing the baby's arms in the front. Only premature babies are swaddled this way, and only until their due date.
- Make sure the blanket you use is large enough and not too heavy.
- If the baby has flushed or red skin, is sweating, or has other signs of being too warm, remove any clothes other than the diaper and swaddle.
- If you are swaddling with a swaddle blanket, follow the instructions for properly wrapping the baby.
- Never swaddle a baby's head or neck, and make sure the baby's breathing is unobstructed.

13.3 Transitioning Out of the Swaddle

Transitioning out of the swaddle might be tricky if the baby isn't ready. The first three months are like a fourth trimester, helping babies slowly adjust to life outside the womb. Some babies stay swaddled for 3 to 7 months. Watch the baby's signals, as some might be ready by the third month.

Here are signs to look for:

- If they struggle in the swaddle all the time and sleep better when they break out.
- If they roll over from their back to their tummy while swaddled.

If you notice these signs, talk to the mom and check if it's okay to stop swaddling. You can start by freeing one arm and see how the baby reacts. If they still startle and wake themselves up, it's too early. Try again in a few weeks. You're on the right track if the baby uses the free arm for comfort. Once both arms are out, you can keep the swaddle around the chest longer. You can remove the wrap altogether when you feel it's the right time.

You can also stop the swaddle suddenly. It might be challenging for a night or two, but the baby will adjust quickly.

There are various transition swaddling blankets and sleep sacks available. For example, Merlin's Magic Sleep Suit is a one-piece suit designed for babies ready to move on from swaddling. It provides a cozy feeling for better sleep but should only be used when sleeping on the back in the crib.

13.4 What to Watch for When Swaddling

Hip Dysplasia

After the birth and for the first few weeks, the baby will be in natural fetal position with legs curled and the arms near the body. Later in development, the legs will straighten. For proper development, the legs must be allowed to straighten and bend with the hips freely mobile. Forcing the legs straight increases the risk of hip dysplasia; if the baby is swaddled too tightly, it can cause this result.

Swaddling and Plagiocephaly

One perceived negative effect of swaddling is flattening of the head or plagiocephaly. Swaddling does not worsen plagiocephaly, but because it is caused by back sleeping and swaddling requires back sleep, it is seen as a cause. (Read more about plagiocephaly in Chapter 18.)

Swaddling and Sudden Infant Death Syndrome (SIDS)

Because the cause of SIDS is unknown, there have been numerous studies done on whether swaddling contributes to the deaths. The research suggests that when the swaddle is done correctly, and the baby is placed on its back to sleep, the advantages of swaddling dramatically outweigh the risks since the infant cannot turn over on their stomach. Never place a swaddled baby on their stomach!

Temperature Regulation

In overly warm instances, swaddled babies can overheat, putting the baby at risk of brain damage or even death. If the baby is sweating, it's time to swaddle in a diaper and a light wrap. While swaddling can be a good way to keep a newborn warm and cozy, skin-to-skin contact is the best way to regulate an infant's temperature.

Sleeping More, Nursing Less

If the mother is breastfeeding, a baby should not be swaddled during feeding time, allowing better access to the breast. Additionally, swaddled babies fall asleep more easily when feeding, making feeding more difficult.

Sensory Stimuli

Sensory stimulus refers to babies learning to organize, which is essential for brain development. During the baby's wake time, it is an excellent time to unswaddle and allow or guide them to put their hands in front of their face. This "centering" organizes their senses. However, return to the swaddle for a good, sound sleep, eliminating the startle reflex caused by the baby's arms being free and waking themselves up.

Chapter 14: Kangaroo Care

Kangaroo Care is a method for all babies, especially preemies, involving three things:

- Skin-to-skin contact
- Breastfeeding only
- Psychological and physical well-being of newborn and mother

During skin-to-skin contact, the baby is tied to the mother's chest with a cloth. The baby wears only a diaper, and the mother wears a shirt or gown with an opening in the front. This contact helps the baby's breathing and brain development. Fathers can also do skin-to-skin. It's beneficial from birth and can be done anytime in the first few weeks, day or night.

Skin-to-skin has various benefits:

- Accelerates brain development, leading to better sleep.
- Reduces stress (lower cortisol levels) and makes the baby cry less.
- Helps regulate body temperature, especially for premature babies.
- Boosts the baby's immune system through contact with the mother's skin.
- Restores the baby's digestive system balance after one hour of skin-to-skin.
- Simulates the womb experience, making the baby feel secure.
- Regulates heart rate and breathing naturally.

Immediate skin-to-skin after birth increases the likelihood of successful breastfeeding. Studies show that skin-to-skin is better than an incubator, especially for smaller babies. Depriving babies of skin-to-skin can lead to issues like ADD, colic, and sleep disorders.

A recent study found that 82% of neonatal intensive care units in the United States use kangaroo care. Pre-term infants experiencing kangaroo care sleep longer, gain more weight, cry less, stay alert longer, and leave the hospital earlier.

Chapter 15: Feeding the Baby

15.1 Breastfeeding

Breastfeeding is considered by many to be the best way to feed a newborn. As a Newborn Care Specialist, your role is to support the mother in her choice and provide information to help her make an informed decision. This section will give information and tips on how to assist the mother and baby if breastfeeding.

Benefits of Breast Milk

- Breast milk adapts to the baby's needs based on their saliva information.
- Contains components that kill cancerous cells, reduce inflammation, act as painkillers, and include stem cells.
- Regulates the baby's temperature and adjusts for twins separately.

The Milk Production Process

The breasts adjust production to the baby's needs during feeding. The more a baby nurses and effectively removes milk from the breasts, the more milk the breasts will produce. If the baby wants more, they'll nurse longer, signaling the breasts to make more milk.

If the mother ever needs to increase the milk supply, empty the breasts thoroughly at each feeding, offer both sides, and pump if needed. The goal is to keep the breasts as empty as possible throughout the day to increase milk production.

There are three stages of milk production:

1. **Colostrum:** Produced during pregnancy and available in the first 36-72 hours after birth, colostrum is the first milk produced by a mother's breasts. Colostrum helps the baby pass stools and prevents jaundice. It has less fat but more carbohydrates, protein, and antibodies to keep the baby healthy. Even though it's low in volume, it's highly nutritious. Colostrum is yellowish-orange, thick, and sticky. A baby usually takes about 2 teaspoons at each feeding.

2. **Transitional Milk:** Creamy white milk that comes after colostrum. It can start as early as twelve hours after birth or within 3 to 10 days. It's similar to colostrum but has more calories and protein and can last 7 to 14 days.
3. **Mature Milk:** Begins 10 to 15 days after birth. It's 90% water, which is crucial for keeping the baby hydrated. The remaining 10% includes carbohydrates, proteins, and fats needed for growth and energy. There are two types:

- Fore-milk: Found at the beginning of the feeding, it's bluish-white and lower in fat and calories.
- Hind-milk: Follows fore-milk, richer and higher in fat. It provides most of the nutrients for the baby's growth and satisfies hunger.

While the concentration of antibodies decreases as it transitions to mature milk in the first two weeks, breast milk keeps providing protection against viruses and bacteria.

Now, let's talk about how much a newborn's stomach can hold:

- A 1-day-old baby's stomach is about 5-7 ml, like the size of a marble.
- By day 3, it grows to about 0.75-1 oz, like a "shooter" marble.
- Around day 7, it's about 1.5-2 oz, like a Ping-Pong ball.

Babies spit up extra milk because their stomachs don't stretch in the early days.

Comfortable Breastfeeding

Positioning is crucial for comfortable breastfeeding. The key is finding a position that works for both the mother and baby—comfort, effectiveness, and the baby gaining enough weight matter most.

One common problem for moms and babies is figuring out the right way to position and latch on. Breastfeeding should not be painful! If a mom and baby are positioned and latched on correctly, breastfeeding should be satisfying. If not, it can lead to sore nipples, cracking, bleeding, and pain for the mom. As an NCS, providing helpful guidance on positioning and unbiased breastfeeding advice is crucial for a positive breastfeeding experience.

Here are simple guidelines for the best feeding experience:

- Lay the baby on their side with good body support, preferably using a pillow.
- Make sure the baby's mouth is level with the nipple.
- The nipple should go straight into the baby's mouth without being pulled out of shape.
- The baby should be held so close that their nose touches the breast during feeding.
- Lips should be curled back, sucking on the breast, not "chewing" on the nipple.
- The tongue should be under the nipple, not on the roof of the mouth.

- If the mom is sitting, avoid leaning too far backward or forward. Pillows can provide extra comfort and support. Putting feet on a stool or low table slightly raises the legs, helping support the baby for a correct latch.

The Perfect Latch

- Use the "C" hold, pressing the breast with the thumb and fingers.
- Ensure the baby's mouth opens wide before inserting the nipple.
- Guide the baby's mouth with a teasing motion if needed.
- Aim the nipple toward the roof of the baby's mouth; the baby's chin should touch the breast first.
- Lips flanged outward during latch.

Sitting Breastfeeding Positions

- Cradle Hold: Baby's head rests on mom's forearm, lying chest to chest.
- Football or Clutch Hold: Hold the baby like carrying a football, allowing visibility.
- Transitional or Cross Cradle Hold: Helpful for monitoring breastfeeding difficulties.
- Lying Down Hold: Suitable for post-cesarean birth or when mom needs to rest.

Reclining Breastfeeding Position

A simpler way to breastfeed is by allowing the mom to recline, like watching TV. Place the baby across the mother's rib cage, with the baby's butt under her opposite breast or supported by her side or over the shoulder. This should be done skin-to-skin initially.

- Ensure the baby's entire body rests against the mother's body.
- Use arms to support the baby comfortably.
- The baby will lift their head and use arms and legs to find the nipple
- Some babies may need gentle guidance.
- Remember, finding the correct position for you and the baby takes practice.

Increasing Comfort for the Mother

- Nurse at the baby's earliest feeding cues for patience and cooperation.
- Apply expressed milk or purified lanolin to moisturize and protect sore nipples.
- Use breast shells to prevent clothing from touching sore nipples.
- Seek help from lactation consultants for persistent issues.

How to Tell if the Baby is Getting Milk

- Observe vigorous nursing for at least 15 minutes on each breast.
- Check for a continual suck, suck, suck, swallow action.
- Feel the mother's breast soften as it empties.
- No clicking sounds in the infant's mouth.
- The mother feels gentle tugging but no pain.

Simple & Smart Breastfeeding Tips

- Change the diaper before or in the middle of the feed to avoid waking a sleeping baby.
- Ensure mom and baby are comfortable during the potentially lengthy feeding process.
- Continue feeding until the baby is satisfied, even if they fall asleep and you have to wake them.

Tips for Large-Breasted Mothers

- Use a rolled towel or washcloth under the breast for support.
- Wear a supportive nursing bra during breastfeeding.
- Tie a stretchy scarf around the neck and under the breast for adjustable support.
- Consider the asymmetrical latch technique for comfortable breastfeeding, which involves lifting the baby's nose further off the breast, off-center, as opposed to centered on the nipple.

How to Awaken a Baby for Breastfeeding

- Undress the baby to allow warmth from mom's breast.
- Massage or rub various body parts like ears, feet, head, palm, belly, spine, or arms.
- Change the baby's position and diaper or engage in activities like sit-ups.
- Lay the baby on the bed without swaddling or use a cool washcloth.
- Lay the baby on the floor unswaddled in front of Mom; baby will start turning side-to-side and wake up.
- Brighten the room.

How Often and How Long to Breastfeed

- Initially, nursing takes 20-45 minutes, decreasing as both mom and baby gain experience.
- During the first week or two, nurse 8-12 times every 24 hours to establish breastfeeding.

Calories for Breastfeeding

- A non-pregnant woman needs about 2,200 calories.
- For breastfeeding a singleton, aim for approximately 2,700 calories.
- Adjust calorie intake based on the number of babies being breastfed.

Identifying the Need for More Frequent Feeding

- Weight loss of more than 10% from birth.
- Poor urine output.
- Prolonged inadequate breastfeeding (three or more times).
- High bilirubin levels (requires pediatrician's evaluation).

Moms Who Want to Nurse and Pump

- Use a commercial breast pump once milk comes in to ease engorgement and establish a nighttime milk supply.
- Alternate breastfeeding and pumping on different breasts to match the baby's needs.
- Consider lactation support in tincture form if experiencing difficulties.
- Express fat-rich morning milk for night feedings.

Power Pumping

- A technique to mimic a baby's frequent nursing during a growth spurt to increase milk supply.
- Involves alternating pumping and resting sessions for about an hour each day.
- It can be concentrated in a power-pumping weekend for faster results.

Frequency of Pumping

- Pump every two hours around the clock for a few days to increase supply.
- Ensure at least 20 minutes per pumping session, possibly extending to 45 minutes to an hour.
- Power pumping can be done for an hour once a day or concentrated in a power pumping weekend.

Storage Time for Human Milk

					Room Temperature	Room Temperature
	Deep Freeze (QOF/ -18°C)	Refrigera-tor Freezer (variable 0°F/-18°C)	Refrigerator (39°F/4°C)	Cooler with Ice Packs Frozen (59°F/1 5°C)	(66°F- 72°F) (19°C- 22°C)	(72°F- 79°F) (22°C- 26°C)
Fresh	Up to 12 months	3-4 months	8 days	24 hours	6-10 hours	4 hours
Frozen, Thawed in Fridge	Do not re-freeze	Do not re-freeze	24 hours	Do not store	4 hours	4 hours
Thawed, Warmed, Not Fed	Do not re-freeze	Do not re-freeze	4 hours	Do not store	Until feeding ends	Until feeding ends
Warmed, Fed	Discard	Discard	Discard	Discard	Until feeding ends	Until feeding ends

Choosing a Container

To store milk in the fridge or freezer, you can use:

- Hard plastic or glass containers with secure lids.
- Freezer milk bags made for storing human milk.
- Avoid using disposable bottle liners.

Warming the Milk

Thaw or heat the milk under warm, running water. Don't let the milk boil. It's normal for stored milk to separate into cream and milk layers. Before checking the temperature, gently swirl the milk to mix in the cream. Don't use a microwave to heat human milk. Do not shake a bottle with breastmilk.

Thawing Milk

If frozen milk has been thawed, you can refrigerate it for up to 24 hours for later use. Don't refreeze it. It's uncertain whether milk left in the bottle after a feeding can be safely kept until the next feeding or should be thrown away.

Bottle Feeding a Breastfed Baby

Breastfeeding is a special time for mom and baby, but sometimes situations arise where using a bottle becomes necessary. This can happen if mom needs a break, goes back to work, or during emergencies. If a baby is used to breastfeeding, introducing a bottle might be challenging, but it can be done.

Here are some tips:

- Introduce Early: Introducing a breast milk bottle within the first week is helpful, even though lactation specialists might suggest otherwise.
- This doesn't harm breastfeeding but allows Mom a break and lets Dad bond with the baby.
- Troubleshooting Tips:
  - Have the mother wear the bottle nipple in her bra for a day to make it smell like her.
  - Put a little milk on the outside of the bottle nipple.
  - Try feeding in a different position, like using a bouncy seat or car seat.
  - Pace feeding.
  - Have your partner feed the baby in another room or when you're away.
  - Feed the bottle in the morning or at night, letting Dad handle this feed.
- Be Patient: Some babies might initially resist the bottle, but they won't starve themselves.
- Keep trying every day and remain consistent with your approach.
- Different Approaches:
  - Serve the bottle at different temperatures.
  - Try different bottle types, nipples, and holding positions.
  - Try pace feeding.
  - Be consistent with the person offering the bottle and the type of bottle.
  - Vary the routine so the baby gets used to the bottle at different times.
- Relax and Stay Calm: Babies can sense your emotions, so try to remain calm and relaxed during bottle-feeding attempts. It's essential not to force the baby but to be gentle yet firm.
- Remember, the key is persistence and finding what works best for your baby.

Nipple Confusion

- Occurs when the baby is introduced to more than one nipple type and becomes confused.
- Signs include refusal to latch, shaking the head, and frustration during feeding.
- Avoid nipple confusion by introducing a bottle early and not offering a pacifier 15 minutes before breastfeeding.

Breastfeeding Issues

When it has normal fullness, the breast and dark area around the nipple stay soft, and milk flows well. Here are possible issues that can arise when breastfeeding:

Engorgement

Engorgement usually starts 2-6 days after birth and goes away in 12-48 hours with proper treatment. The breast gets bigger and hard, the skin stretches, and it might feel warm, tender, or throbbing. Sometimes, there's a low-grade fever.

Can happen:

- In the areola or breast body.
- In one or both breasts.
- Building to a peak, staying the same, or peaking multiple times.

How to handle this:

- Feed the baby early and often, at least ten times a day.
- Use a pump if needed, making sure to empty the breasts.
- Feed on the baby's schedule. Wake them every 3 hours during the day. Let them sleep 4-5 hours at night after the baby has regained their birthweight. Always have the pediatrician's approval first.
- Let the baby finish one breast before switching sides.
- Massage the breasts gently before and during nursing.
- Use cool compresses for 20 minutes before nursing.

Treatment:

- Use warmth for a few minutes before nursing.
- If latching is problematic, express or pump for a few minutes before nursing.
- Use cold compresses (ice packs over cloth) between feedings for 20 minutes on and 20 minutes off.

Tips for Treating Sore Nipples

After nursing:

- Express a few drops of milk and massage into the nipples for healing.
- Keep nipples dry after feedings.
- Expose nipples to sunlight for a few minutes (but not too much!).

- Avoid using soap on nipples; nipples have natural oils.
- Check your bra; make sure it's not too tight or rough.
- If too tender, use breast shells in your bra to keep fabric away.
- Consider Medela gel pads for soreness but only for the first week, not for cracked or bleeding nipples.

Candida Infection on Nipples (Thrush)

Candida is a highly contagious fungus that likes warm, dark, and moist places. It can be found in various body parts like the mouth, vagina, diaper area, skin folds, and sometimes on nipples. **Note: After taking antibiotics, Candida is common.**

Suspect Candida if:

- Nipples are very sore, burning, itching, red, or blistered.
- Mom feels sharp pains in the breasts during or after feeding.
- Standard remedies for sore nipples don't work.
- Baby has oral thrush or a yeasty diaper rash.
- Nipples suddenly become sore after pain-free breastfeeding.

Tips for Candida Relief

Have the mother do the following:

- Expose nipples to sunlight for a few minutes several times a day.
- Air-dry nipples after each feeding.
- Avoid plastic-lined breast pads; change pads after each feeding.
- Wear 100% cotton bras and wash them daily in hot water.
- Wash pump parts in a bleach solution and boil daily.

Treating Candida Infection on the Nipple

- Eat yogurt with live active cultures and take oral acidophilus.
- Apply yogurt to your breasts to kill any yeast.
- Use a solution of 1 teaspoon baking soda mixed with 1 cup of water on affected areas.
- Apply an anti-fungal cream (prescribed by a doctor) on nipples, making sure to wash it off before nursing.

Plugged Milk Ducts

Sometimes, a milk duct gets blocked, causing a tender lump beneath the nipple. To prevent infection:

- Continue breastfeeding on the affected side. A baby has strong sucking capabilities and will drain the duct when you help the mom position the lower lip where the duct is clogged.
- Breastfeed on the affected side first.
- Vary baby's position for complete milk duct drainage.
- Apply moist heat before feeding.
- Rest and nurse in bed.

Take oral granular lecithin or lecithin capsules daily to prevent plugged ducts from reoccurring.

Mastitis

Mastitis means the breast is inflamed, causing pain, redness, and swelling. Signs include:

- Intense pain, heat, tenderness, redness, and swelling in part or all of the breast.
- Feeling tired, achy, and having chills or flu-like symptoms.
- Fever of 101°F or higher.

Preventing Mastitis

Relieve engorgement promptly, breastfeed frequently, and avoid compressing breasts against the mattress.

Treating Mastitis

- Drink fluids and rest.
- Follow engorgement rules.
- Boost the immune system with good nutrition.
- Continue nursing to prevent a breast infection from turning into an abscess.
- Apply heat before and ice after nursing.
- Massage the duct while nursing.

- Drink plenty of water.
- Use raw garlic, cabbage leaves, Vitamin C, probiotics, and fermented cod liver oil.

Foods to Avoid When Breastfeeding

This list is for ANY baby with ANY digestion issues, gas, reflux, crying, etc.

Dairy

Vegetables

- Broccoli
- Cabbage
- Cauliflower
- Tomato Juice
- Cucumber
- Garlic
- Rhubarb
- Green Peppers
- Brussels Sprouts
- Tomato
- Corn
- Onions
- Turnips
- Kale and lettuce (salad is one of the big offenders although spinach seems fine)

Fruits

- Apple (especially peels)
- Bananas (can cause constipation)
- Citrus fruits
- Figs
- Coconut

Drinks

- Dairy of any kind is a huge offender (lactose intolerance can provoke reflux in some babies)
- Coffee (even decaffeinated)
- Tea
- Carbonated or caffeinated beverages

Other Miscellaneous

- Beans
- Tofu (in large quantities)
- Fatty or Fried Foods (fats take longer to digest)
- Chocolate
- Black pepper
- Oats (rolled oats are OK)
- Chili powder
- Vinegar
- Honey
- Creamy food such as gravy, etc. (basically with a high fat content)

Baby Breastfeeding Challenges

- High or unusually shaped palate
- Short tongue or receding chin
- Attached frenulum
- Difficulty recognizing hunger cues
- Jaundice

Is Breastfeeding the Right Choice?

Breastfeeding can offer many benefits for both the baby and the mother. However, it may not be the best option for everyone. Here are some of the potential pros and cons of breastfeeding:

Pros of breastfeeding

- **Provides the ideal nutrition for the baby:** Breast milk is specifically designed to meet the nutritional needs of infants, and it contains antibodies and other substances that can help protect the baby against infection and illness.
- **Helps with bonding:** The skin-to-skin and eye contact involved in breastfeeding can promote bonding between the mother and the baby.
- **May reduce the risk of certain health problems:** Breastfeeding has been associated with a lower risk of certain health problems in both the mother and the baby, such as allergies, asthma, ear infections, and some types of cancer.
- **Convenient and cost-effective:** Breast milk is always available at the right temperature and doesn't require any preparation or equipment. Breastfeeding is also usually less expensive than formula feeding.

Cons of breastfeeding

- **May be difficult and uncomfortable:** Breastfeeding can be challenging for some mothers, particularly in the first few weeks, and it may cause soreness, engorgement, or other discomfort.
- **Can be time-consuming:** Breastfeeding can require a significant time commitment, especially in the early weeks and months.
- **Can limit the mother's freedom:** Because breastfeeding requires the mother to be physically present and available to the baby, it can limit her ability to go out or engage in other activities.
- **Can be emotionally demanding:** Breastfeeding can be emotionally demanding for some mothers, and it may contribute to feelings of exhaustion, frustration, or guilt if they are not able to breastfeed as long as they hoped.

It's important to note that there are ways to address many of the challenges associated with breastfeeding, and there are also alternatives to breastfeeding, such as formula feeding. Ultimately, the decision to breastfeed is personal and should be based on individual circumstances and preferences.

15.2 Bottle Feeding

There are so many new and expensive bottles to choose from; how do you know which is the best? We always recommend using products that do not use the organic compound Bisphenol A (BPA). In the past, many plastic products such as baby bottles, plastic plates and cutlery, storage containers, and drink bottles have been made using BPA. Over the years, concerns have been raised about its effects on human health, especially when used in food contact materials and articles. Many jurisdictions worldwide now regulate the use of BPA.

Our favorite and most recommended BPA-free nipples and bottles are the Dr. Browns, which have wide and narrow nipples. They seem to do best with not allowing as much air into the nipple as other bottles do. Most of the time, families buy expensive bottles and end up changing over to Dr. Brown's. Some people want to avoid Dr. Brown bottles because they have so many little parts, but we have found they work well.

How to Prepare the Formula

Each family is different. Some families will choose to feed their baby with cold formula. Some may choose to warm the formula. Make sure it's not too hot. Some people think room temperature is the best, as it takes the least time to prepare. It's important to note that all poweder formulat has bacteria; as a result, the water needs to be boiled before mixing. The formula can then be refrigerated and used throughout the next 24 hours.

1. Boil water (microwaving is not recommended because it changes the water molecules and formula nutrients)
2. Add the desired amount of water to the bottle.
3. Add the formula and mix well.
4. Refrigerate to cool the formula to the desired temperature.
5. To warm the bottle later, place it in the bottle warmer or a pan of hot water and leave it until it reaches the desired temperature.

Bottle Nipples

It is important to find the right fit of nipple for each baby. There are breastfed babies that need the wider nipple and there are babies that just like smaller ones. The nipple is dependent on the bottle that you choose. There are latex, rubber, and silicone nipples. Some bottle manufacturers make both the rubber and the silicone for you to choose from.

Which material is best for the baby? Latex nipples are soft and the most flexible of the three choices. They are also not as durable. Rubber lasts longer but is less flexible. Silicone is the firmest and, as a result, holds its shape longer. Silicone also lasts longer, which is one reason why they cost more.

The shape of the nipples varies as well:

- Standard nipples: rounded tip and easy for baby to use
- Flat-topped orthodontic: the flat top is designed to accommodate the baby's palate and gums; they mimic the shape and flexibility of the mother's nipple, which is good if the mother is breastfeeding and bottle feeding the baby.
- Nubbin nipples that elongate: short, flattened tips; if the baby sucks hard enough and the mouth is open enough, the tip will elongate during sucking.
- Tri-cut nipples: longer than the standard, which releases milk farther into the baby's mouth, making it easier to swallow

You will need to increase the size of the nipple hole as the baby grows. We start with the newborn, then at a month old, we typically go to the number one nipple, and at the third month, we usually go to the number two nipple, but all of this varies according to the manufacturer of the nipple.

The way to know if the nipple size is too small is if it takes over 30 minutes for the baby to finish the amount of milk they normally drink. Baby formula should drip approximately one drop per second. On the other hand, if the baby chokes or the mouth fills fast, the hole may be too large.

When you increase the nipple size, you want to position the baby with his head up higher, almost in a sitting position, so that he can adjust. If the milk is coming out too fast, lower the bottle and adjust it so the baby can acclimate to the new flow.

If the nipple looks discolored, thin, cracked, or worn, replace it. Always wash with soap and water before the first use.

Sterilizing the Bottle

Some mothers sterilize the bottles before every use. However, it doesn't need to be done so often. It is enough to wash them in hot, soapy water with a baby-safe soap. There are three times critical for sterilizing:

- When the bottles are first purchased, use a sterilizer and dryer or boil them for five minutes, then let them air dry.
- If the baby has a yeast infection or thrush, sterilize after every use for two weeks AFTER the infection is gone.
- If the water system is on a private well.

Feeding Schedule

There are three ways people approach feeding a baby:

1. Demand Feeding: Feeding the baby whenever and however much they want. If the baby is fussy, you feed them. If they take a small amount and fall asleep, that's okay. This method can be tiring for the parent, especially if breastfeeding, as the baby decides when to eat. It's a bit easier for bottle-feeding, but night feeding can be unpredictable. Demand Feeding might lead to a baby who always wants to suck for comfort, not just for hunger.
2. Scheduled Feedings: Some parents prefer a set schedule, feeding the baby every 3 hours, no sooner or later. This can be rigid and may overstimulate the baby, leading to fussiness and lack of sleep.
3. Responsible Feeding: This is a compromise between demand and scheduled feeding. Feed the baby every 3 hours, but adjust if the baby needs more. In 7-10 days make efforts to have awake time with playtime and or another means of stimulation. Try to get the baby on a schedule for naps between 9-11 and 1-4, starting around 4-5 months old; the baby will soon conform to the schedule. Expect the baby to self-soothe during these times, which might be tough initially but gets easier over time.

Feeding Schedule Tips

- In the first week after birth, give the baby one to two ounces of infant formula every two to three hours if the baby is only getting infant formula and no breast milk. Give the baby more if he or she is showing signs of hunger. Most infant formula-fed newborns will feed 8 to 12 times in 24 hours.
- Babies gradually eat more during the first month until three to four ounces (90 to 120 ml) per feed, totaling 32 ounces daily. Formula-fed babies typically eat on a more regular schedule every three to four hours. Breastfed babies usually eat smaller, more frequent feedings than formula-fed infants.
- At first, bottle-fed babies can go longer between feeds than breastfed babies; it usually evens out at three to four weeks.
- If the baby sleeps longer than four to five hours at night during the first few weeks after birth and misses feedings, wake them up and offer a bottle.

- **Always check with a pediatrician before stretching the feedings at night.**
- The baby should be fed every three hours during the day. After the baby is sleeping for 12 hours at night (by 12 weeks), you may start stretching out the daytime feedings to four-hour stretches.
- Cluster feed in the early evening.
- Depending on weight, the baby should be able to go four to six hours during the night.
- The baby will consume six to eight ounces (180–240 ml) at each of four or five feedings in 24 hours by five months.

Formula Feeding Based on Body Weight

On average, the baby should take about 2.5 ounces (75 ml) of infant formula daily for every pound (453 g) of body weight. Babies regulate their intake from day to day to meet their specific needs, so let them tell you when they've had enough. They're probably finished if they become fidgety or easily distracted during a feeding. They might still be hungry if they drain the bottle and continue smacking their lips.

There are high and low limits, however. Discuss it with the pediatrician if the baby consistently wants more or less than this. Some babies have higher needs for sucking and may want to suck on a pacifier after feeding.

Guidelines for Weight Gain with Bottle Feeding

In the first few months, babies gain about one ounce (28 grams) daily. That slows down to about 20 grams a day at around four months. As they turn six months old, many babies gain about 10 grams or less daily.

Feeding Guideline Chart

The chart below targets a baby who weighs 6-8 lbs or more at birth. If the baby is premature, reference the chart but adjust it according to the baby's weight.

Age	If Bottle-feeding, how much?	If breastfeeding, how long?	How often?	Comments
First 3 days	1.5-2 oz. every 3 hours (between 15-20 oz. total)	As long as the baby wants to nurse.	Every two to three hours.	Breast-feeding mothers need to feed more often for milk to flow (usually starts the first 3 days).
Up to 6 weeks	2-5 oz. per feed (7-8 feeds per day)	Up to 45 minutes	Every 3 hours during the day. If you cluster feed in the early evening, the baby should be able to sleep 4-6 hours.	Bottle-fed babies can go longer between feeds until it evens out around 3-4 weeks.
6 weeks – 4 months	4-8 oz. per feed.	Up to 30 minutes	Every 3 hours during the day. By 12 weeks, should be able to sleep 12 hours.	After the baby is sleeping for 12 hours at night (by 12 weeks), try stretching out the daytime feedings to every 4 hours.

Is the Baby Eating Enough?

There are several things you can observe to tell if the baby is getting enough milk or formula:

- Is the baby lethargic or less active?
- Does the stomach feel full (hard)?
- Is the baby happy and content?

- Is the baby having at least one bowl movement per day? How many wet and dirty diapers?
- Are the baby's eyes alert and bright?
- Is the skin healthy-looking?
- Does the baby vigorously move its arms and legs?
- Are the baby's nails growing?
- Are development milestones being met?

Signs of Underfeeding

- If the baby is cranky after draining the bottle.
- If the baby is gaining less than ½ pound a week.
- If the baby does not have a wet diaper for each feeding.

Signs of Overfeeding

- Spitting up (this can also be a sign that the formula isn't working for the baby).
- Fussiness and abdominal pain after feeding (this can also be a sign of a bad formula).
- Fast weight gain (over ½ pound per week); if this is the case, feed every three hours or more and offer a pacifier after the bottle (the baby might just have a strong urge to suck and isn't actually hungry).

15.3 Infant Formulas

Breast milk is considered the best and most natural food for infants, as it provides a unique combination of nutrients and antibodies that can support a baby's immune system and overall development. However, for parents who cannot breastfeed, a variety of infant formulas are available that aim to provide complete nutrition and support a baby's health and development.

Infant formula is a specialized food product designed to provide complete nutrition for infants who are not breastfed or who are partially breastfed. Infant formula typically contains a blend of carbohydrates, proteins, and fats, along with essential vitamins and minerals, to support the growth and development of a baby.

Infant formula is available in three forms: powdered, liquid concentrate, and ready-to-use. Powdered formula is the most common form and is easy to store and transport. Liquid concentrate formula requires mixing with water before use, while ready-to-use formula is pre-mixed and requires no additional preparation.

Different infant formula types are available, including cow's-milk-based, soy-based, and specialized formulas for infants with specific dietary needs or health conditions. It is important to consult a healthcare provider before choosing an infant formula for the baby, as they can help determine which formula best suits the baby's needs.

Most Holistic, Healing Infant Formulas

While all infant formulas are required to meet specific nutritional standards, some parents may be interested in formulas that are marketed as more holistic or healing. Here are a few examples:

Organic infant formula: Some parents may prefer organic formulas from ingredients grown without synthetic pesticides or fertilizers. Organic formulas may also be free from certain additives or processing methods some parents may want to avoid.

Goat milk formula: Some parents may choose goat milk-based formulas as an alternative to cow's milk-based formulas. Goat milk has a different composition than cow's milk, and some parents believe is easier for babies to digest.

Probiotic infant formula: Probiotics are beneficial bacteria supporting a healthy gut microbiome. Some infant formulas include probiotics to support digestive health and immune function.

Hydrolyzed protein formula: Some infants may have difficulty digesting certain proteins, such as those found in cow's milk or soy. Hydrolyzed protein formulas are processed in a way that breaks down the proteins into smaller fragments, which may be easier for some infants to digest.

The effectiveness and safety of different types of infant formulas can vary based on a baby's individual needs and health status.

15.4 Burping the Baby

Burping the baby is extremely important and yet, most people do not know how to do it properly. Typically, you will burp the baby in the middle of feeding and at the end. Some babies require more, and you may have to burp every ounce or so of feeding.

The most common burping method is the over-the-shoulder method, placing the head on your shoulder and patting the back. For this method, start at the lower back and move your hand up while patting, then back to the lower back. Start rubbing in circles on the baby's back after patting for a moment. The baby will likely squirm and be restless until the burp comes.

- ➤ A variation is to straddle the baby on your arm with its tummy down and its head on your hand while you rub the back.

- Another method is to sit the baby on your lap with your hand supporting the baby's chest under their chin and then pat the back.
- You can also lay the baby across your lap with the tummy on your leg.
- And finally, a less common method that works for a baby that is hard to burp. Place the baby over your shoulder, hanging its tummy on your shoulder blade. Place your hand on the baby's bottom and move the baby up and down.

Be firm with your pats. Many new parents are afraid they will hurt the baby. If your baby hasn't burped in less than a minute, you will need to be more firm. You will not hurt the baby.

15.5 Pacifiers

Babies are born with a natural desire to suck and many babies suck their thumb in the womb. Sucking is a way of self-soothing and calming their nervous system, which is why pacifiers are sometimes necessary. Many people are afraid to use pacifiers because they think that their baby will have nipple confusion or become dependent on them. Some people believe that if the baby sucks on a pacifier, then they won't want to suck on the mother's breast. In our experience, this rarely happens.

The way to prevent confusion is to make sure that the baby is latching correctly to the mom regularly. Some babies seem to need to suck even after having had a full feed; this is when we would consider using a pacifier. A pacifier is a tool; if used correctly, it can easily be removed when the time is right.

Babies with reflux have an even stronger need to suck since it helps them relieve their burning or discomfort. It is important to know the difference between a strong urge to suck and hunger, and it is important not to overfeed the infant. Below is a list of the pros and cons of using pacifiers that should be considered.

Pros:

- Pacifiers can soothe a fussy baby.
- Pacifiers can help the baby fall asleep when they have difficulty settling down.
- Pacifiers can help distract a hungry baby until their bottle is ready and can be helpful during bathtime or other stressful events.
- Pacifiers may help reduce the risk of SIDS (Sudden Infant Death Syndrome)
- Pacifiers are easy to get rid of when they are no longer needed.

Cons:

- Dental problems can occur with prolonged use.
- It may increase the risk of middle ear infections.

- The baby may become dependent on the pacifier.

Suggestions:

- The most important thing about pacifiers is that you have to keep them clean. Before you use a new pacifier, wash it with soap and water. Most are also dishwasher safe, and can be sterilized easily.
- Use caution when using pacifier clips. Never use a string or strap that is long enough to get caught around the baby's neck.
- Make sure to watch for signs of deterioration and replace the pacifiers often. A worn pacifier can become cracked or torn, be a choking hazard, or harbor bacteria.
- Let the baby set the pace. Offer the pacifier, but if they are not interested, you can try again later. If they fall asleep and the pacifier falls out, there is no need to put it back in.
- Try other ways of calming or soothing the baby like repositioning or patting before offering the pacifier. The time will come when the baby needs to learn to self-soothe without the pacifier.

15.6 Feeding Multiple Babies

When you feed multiple babies, simultaneous feeding is best. Put each baby in the same position every time, like on a blanket on the bed. If they need support, use a rolled-up blanket or a boppy. To keep them on the same schedule, try to feed them together versus separately. Hold one baby on your lap and the other next to your leg when feeding from a sitting position. Hold both bottles or prop one while holding the other, keeping an eye on both to prevent choking. Change and attend to both babies to maintain the same schedule even if one is still sleeping.

To make things easier with multiples, use color codes; assign each baby a color for their bottle rings, pacifiers, etc.

Chapter 16: The Day-to-Day Routine

16.1 Understanding Crying

Crying is a natural emotional response that humans and some animals exhibit in response to various stimuli, such as sadness, pain, joy, or frustration. It is often accompanied by tears, facial expressions, and vocalizations such as sobbing or whimpering.

Crying can serve several purposes, including expressing and releasing emotions, signaling distress or need, and facilitating social connection and support. For example, crying can be a way of expressing sadness and grief over the loss of a loved one, or it can be a way of seeking comfort and support from others when feeling overwhelmed or stressed.

The brain and the nervous system regulate the act of crying. Research has shown that crying can activate the release of various chemicals in the body, such as endorphins and oxytocin, which can help reduce stress and promote feelings of well-being and social bonding.

16.2 Infant Crying

Infant crying is a normal and natural part of development. Crying is the primary way infants communicate their needs and feelings, especially before they can express themselves through language. It is also a way for infants to release tension and stress, essential for their emotional and physical well-being.

Infants may cry for various reasons, such as hunger, discomfort, tiredness, boredom, overstimulation, or illness. Parents and caregivers must be attentive to their infant's cues and respond promptly and appropriately to their cries.

Research suggests that responding sensitively to an infant's cries can help promote a secure attachment between the infant and caregiver, which can have long-term benefits for the infant's social development.

It is also important to note that excessive or inconsolable crying in infants can be a sign of underlying health issues, such as colic, reflux, or infection. If a parent or caregiver is concerned about their infant's crying patterns, they should consult a healthcare provider for guidance and support.

16.3 Crying It Out (CIO)

Crying It Out (CIO) is a technique used to allow babies to self-soothe by crying. While there is some anti-CIO sentiment, in the official journal of the AAP, the conclusion is that "Behavioral sleep techniques have no marked long-lasting effects (positive or negative). Parents and Health professionals can confidently use these techniques to reduce the short-to-medium-term burden of infant sleep problems and maternal depression."

Ongoing childhood stress can have long-term effects, but if a baby is in a loving and harmonious environment, putting a baby down to sleep when they are crying does not require your extended supervision. They might be crying because they are over-tired and need the rest; they might be having a short temper tantrum; it might be because you took them away from playtime. Because crying is the only way they can communicate, you must learn how to understand their crying.

There is an anti-CIO belief that it causes ADHD. However, there is evidence that ADHD is more likely from a sleep-deprived child, which might be linked to when the child was a baby and wasn't taught how to sleep correctly.

It is important to remember that the CIO is not a punishment or a lack of nurturing by the mother. Instead, it is a lesson in self-soothing. It has no reflection on a mother's care for their baby. It is more likely they are telling the parent they want them, not that they need them.

Excessive crying, neglect, or leaving them to cry for extended periods is not recommended. Instead, we encourage you to use the *Joy of Sleep Method*, which we will cover in Chapter 17.

16.4 Soothing Techniques

There are multiple ways to calm a crying baby. Many of the best soothing techniques involve mimicking/recreating environmental conditions similar to the womb.

Dr. Karp's Soothing Technique

Dr. Harvey Karp is an assistant professor of pediatrics at UCLA and a renowned expert on children's health. He describes the first few months of a baby's life as the fourth trimester, in which the baby has difficulty getting used to the large amount of stimuli in the outside world. Dr. Karp developed a soothing technique that he refers to as the "five S's system."

The Five S's

1. **Swaddling:** As previously stated, swaddling is an excellent way to help calm a baby since it provides them with warmth and a feeling of security, similar to how they felt in the womb.
2. **Side/stomach positioning:** Holding the baby on its side can help them with digestion and remind them of being in the womb. If the infant falls asleep, reposition

them on their back for safety. Place the baby on either side while holding them to provide comforting support.

3. **Shushing sounds:** When babies are in the womb, they are used to hearing the sounds of blood circulating through the placenta and the uterus. Shushing sounds imitate the noises in the womb, which helps the baby feel safe and calm. For this reason, infants don't like silence and prefer white noise to calm them. White noise machines are a crucial tool when sleep training a baby.
4. **Swinging:** Swinging motions are calming and comforting to babies. Babies like to be rocked back and forth in a slow, steady motion. Rocking also gives them the comfort of movements they were used to in the womb. Support the infant's head and neck while rocking them back and forth. Infant swings can be a good alternative method of rocking the baby.
5. **Sucking**: Offering a pacifier or a nipple to feed can help soothe a fussy baby. Babies naturally like sucking, and it is an excellent way to get them to stop crying since they can't suck and cry at the same time. Sucking releases natural chemicals that trigger the calming reflex, and they have a profound effect on the nervous system. If the infant doesn't want the pacifier, do not force it on them; try a different soothing method.

Please watch Dr. Karp's video for a more detailed explanation. https://www.youtube.com/watch?v=xRkRlvPGywM&ab_channel=Today%27sParent

16.6 Additional Soothing Techniques

- Hold the baby close to your body while swaddled.
- Walk or sway while holding the baby.
- Hum while holding the baby
- Play calming music or sing a lullaby.
- Rub/massage/pat
- Stand outside in nature.
- Earthing or grounding: When you touch your body to the ground (bare feet on the grass or dirt), it dissipates static electricity and extraneous environmental electrical charges in your body and the baby. www.earthing.com

If these techniques haven't worked, here is something else to try:

- Put the baby in the crib and allow the baby to cry for a few minutes

- Take a break and ask Mom for help if needed
- Take deep breaths and relax
- Reassess if all the baby's needs have been met

Chapter 17: Scheduling a Baby for Optimal Sleep

This section discusses the importance of sleep and sleep training to the health of the baby.

17.1 The Importance of Sleep

There are three significant reasons for optimal sleep:

- **Body Maturation:** Sleep is a fundamental physiological need for physical recovery, body growth, learning, and memory. Chronic sleep deprivation can lead to exhaustion, physical damage, immune system dysfunction, severe stress, and death. The growth hormone, crucial for a baby's physical growth, is mainly secreted during deep sleep. Severe sleep disorders may result in inadequate hormone secretion and compromised body maturation.
- **Brain Growth:** Active behavior during sleep, such as uneven breathing, darting eyes, smiling, and grimacing, indicates Rapid Eye Movement (REM) sleep—a stage associated with dreaming. Babies spend about 50% of their sleep in REM sleep, essential for brain maturation, learning, and development. A baby is born with around 30% of their full brain size, and in the first three years, the brain grows rapidly. REM sleep facilitates information processing. Disruptions to REM sleep may compromise learning.
- **Time to Sleep:** Insufficient or disrupted sleep makes babies agitated, nervous, hyperactive, and hard to manage. These signs signal when a baby is ready for sleep. Missing the sleep window can make it challenging for the baby to calm down and fall asleep. Babies, like adults, have an internal biological clock, making it easier to sleep at certain times. Maintaining a regular schedule and consistent bedtime helps regulate the biological clock, fostering healthy sleep patterns for the baby and parents.

17.2 Tips for Scheduling Optimal Sleep

Establishing a sleep schedule for a newborn can be challenging. Here are some tips for scheduling a newborn for optimal sleep patterns:

- **Follow the baby's cues:** Watch for the baby's cues that they are tired, such as rubbing their eyes or yawning, and put them down for a nap before they get overtired.
- **Create a consistent routine:** Newborns thrive on consistency. Establish a bedtime routine, such as bathing, feeding, and a lullaby, so the baby knows it's time to sleep.
- **Create a calm sleep environment:** Make sure the baby's sleep environment is quiet and peaceful. Use a white noise machine to block out background noise and ensure the room is dark. Swaddling the baby can also help them feel secure.
- **Limit stimulation:** Newborns can become overstimulated quickly, making it hard for them to fall asleep. Limit the baby's exposure to bright lights or loud noises before bedtime.
- **Gradually increase awake time:** As the baby gets older, progressively increase their awake time between naps. This will help them naturally establish a more regular sleep schedule.
- **Be patient:** Remember every baby is different, and establishing a sleep schedule may take some time. Be patient, and try different strategies until you find what works best for the baby.

17.3 Understanding Sleep and Sleep Issues for the Newborn Infant

Sleep Patterns: Newborns do not have a well-established sleep pattern. They sleep for 16 or more hours a day, but this sleep is in short periods, usually two to four hours before they wake up to eat, have their diaper changed, or be comforted. They may also have periods of alertness and activity during the day, making it harder for them to settle down for sleep at night.

Sleep Cycles: Newborns have a shorter sleep cycle than adults, lasting only 50 to 60 minutes. This means that they move between light sleep and deep sleep more frequently. As a result, they wake up more often and need to be soothed back to sleep.

Sleep Environment: The newborn's sleep environment should be safe and comfortable. The baby should sleep on their back on a firm, flat surface without any pillows, blankets, or toys in the crib. The room should be kept at 68-72 degrees F., not too hot or too cold. Keeping the room dark and quiet, with minimal stimulation, is also important.

Sleep Issues: Newborns may experience sleep issues such as colic, reflux, or sleep apnea. Colic is a condition where the baby cries for more than three hours a day, three days a week, for at least three weeks. Reflux is a condition where the baby spits up frequently and experiences discomfort. Sleep apnea is when the baby stops breathing for short periods during sleep.

Parents should consult with a healthcare professional for any concerns about sleep issues.

17.4 Teaching Self-Soothing

Self-soothing is a method designed to help the baby learn and develop independently without constant attention. For many reasons, learning to self-soothe is crucial to a baby's development, but it is critical for sleep training. Here are some self-soothing tips:

- Approach without emotions. Follow the mantra, "I cannot fix it for you, but I will go through it with you, by your side." Children thrive with consistency, boundaries, and love.
- Teaching a baby to self-soothe is challenging for most parents, especially if it's their first child. Let the parent know that once the baby learns, they can put themselves to sleep. It's crucial to let the child figure this out on their own as the sleep habits established early will support them as they grow.
- Start the self-soothing technique during the daytime so the child is familiar with it at night. Start working on this process from two to three weeks of age.
- At two to four weeks, let the baby fuss if you are sure they are fed, changed, burped, and sleepy. Allow them to fuss for up to three minutes before intervening with one of the following:
    - Change the baby's position
    - Offer pacifier
    - Pick the baby up, pat a couple of times, and put them right back down.
    - Consoling where they lay is recommended over picking up, unless crying is out of control.
    - Shushing them
- If the baby stops crying for 15 seconds or more within the 3-minute period, restart the time.
- If the baby stops crying only to start again with an accelerated cry, you may pick them up, pat them, and put them back down when settled.
- When using this method, avoid talking to the baby or making eye contact. Let the baby self-soothe without interference or attention.
- Leave the room as soon as the baby calms down.

Remember, your role is to assist the baby in calming down but not to fix their problems or soothe them back to sleep. They need to learn this process independently. Starting this method after four weeks may take a bit longer, but consistency brings significant benefits long term.

17.5 What is SleepTraining?

Sleep training is teaching your baby to go from being awake to falling asleep without needing outside assistance, without needing to be fed right before sleep, and without needing to be rocked or held. Sleep training starts after the infant is at least 12 weeks or 12 pounds. However, sleep *conditioning* takes place from day one by scheduling awake, sleep, and feed times, and monitoring the amount of food.

There are two things we cannot do for children: eat for them and sleep for them. Therefore, teaching them to eat and sleep healthily is essential, especially when they are infants. Children not taught early the skill of self-soothing (see above)—a necessary tool of sleep training—may have trouble sleeping as toddlers and adults.

Sleep training is not just about making life easier for the parents; it's about providing the infant's basic needs. Here are tips to keep in mind:

- Create a clear plan for sleep training that differs from sleep conditioning. Ensure both you and the parents are ready practically and emotionally before starting.
- Practical preparations involve considering the parents' schedule, avoiding starting the plan when they are busy or have visitors.
- Discuss and agree on the plan with the parents, ensuring mutual understanding and support. Being on the same page prevents issues when parents take over on weekends.
- Consistency is crucial once the plan is launched. Stick to it for a couple of weeks unless the baby isn't ready, and a temporary pause is needed. Resisting the urge to give in during challenging moments is essential to avoid starting over.
- Be prepared to lose some sleep during the Cry-It-Out (CIO) phase. Start on a night when missing some sleep won't be a problem. Anticipate difficult nights, and remember that the short-term challenge leads to improved sleep for everyone in the household.
- Adapt the method to suit the family. If the chosen approach feels too harsh, consider a more gradual method that aligns with the family's comfort level.

17.6 Sleep Training Methods

There are many approaches to sleep training. Our favorites are the following two, but we briefly discuss other approaches as well.

Joy of Sleep Method

The Joy of Sleep is the ideal method for sleep training when the baby comes in as a blank slate. This method establishes a daily routine early to set the foundation for the baby to learn self-soothing, while giving them a feeling of predictability that allows them to feel safe. Some parents wait for the baby to tell them what is next, but our job is to anticipate and meet the need before the baby gets stressed, overtired, or over-hungry. If you can help them understand the pattern by immediately establishing a routine in which you anticipate their needs, then there is no reason for crying.

The Joy of Sleep is a no-cry approach and must be started within the first month of life since this is when you can easily teach good habits. Each family is provided a daily schedule customized according to their routine and the baby's specific needs. I have used this method for over 20 years and now call it **The Joy of Sleep Method** because it has been so effective. This method works for singletons, twins, triplets, and more.

The **Joy of Sleep Method** training seminar provides a more detailed explanation of this approach.

Nap Training Method

Nap Training is a method we use for babies 12 weeks of age or older who have not been taught the **Joy of Sleep Method**. This method teaches the baby self-soothing techniques during naps since these are shorter sleep intervals. **The Joy of Sleep Method** training seminar provides a more detailed explanation of the Nap training approach.

Other Sleep Training Methods

- **Slow Gentle Method (Reducing Feeding)**
  - Gradually reduce the amount of milk offered by 1 ounce every 4th day, substituting with water.
  - Continue until feeding the baby about an ounce of water only.
- **Controlled Crying Method**
  - NCS goes in every 10 minutes to pat or talk to the baby, not picking them up.
  - Extend intervals gradually each night.

- **Camping Out Method**
  - Put baby down awake, place a chair beside the crib, and shush the baby.
  - Gradually move the chair further away until the baby falls asleep without you in the room.
- **Pick Up Put Down Method**
  - Pick up and settle the baby when they fuss, put them down when calm.
  - Consistent use may complete within a week to 10 days.
- **Rock-A-Bye Method**
  - Gradual process of reducing rocking until the baby can self-settle.
  - Requires commitment and consistency over several days.
- **Ferber Method**
  - Controlled crying with increasing wait times each night.
  - No picking up, only patting on the back.
- **CIO Method (Cry It Out)**
  - Fast and easy method for babies over 10-12 weeks.
  - Check for basic needs, offer a pacifier, let the baby cry for 30-45 minutes.
  - Gradual improvement over a week to ten days.

Note: Each method has variations and may take time for the baby to adjust. Parents should choose a method they can commit to and be consistent with. If the baby is over 12 weeks, a more strict approach may be necessary for quicker results. It's crucial to avoid giving in to crying to prevent setbacks in the sleep training process.

Training a Consistent Wake-Up Time

To set a consistent wake-up time for a baby at 10-12 weeks:

1. Aim for the desired wake-up time, e.g., 8 a.m.
2. If the baby wakes earlier, soothe them without feeding until the target time.
3. Gradually extend the wait time each day until reaching the goal.
4. Be consistent, even if setbacks occur, and avoid early feedings less than 1 hour before the target time.

Wake to Sleep

For babies waking up prematurely during naps or mornings:

1. Gently rouse the baby one hour before expected waking and aid in transitioning back to sleep.
2. This helps create new neural pathways and encourages longer sleep.

Sleep Training an 8-Month-Old

1. Establish a bedtime routine.
2. Put the baby in their bed and let them cry for short intervals.
3. Gradually increase wait times.
4. Be mindful of separation anxiety.
5. Consistency is crucial; avoid rewarding crying.

Sleep Training a 1-Year-Old

1. Follow a consistent bedtime routine.
2. Introduce comfort objects but remove sleep aids like bottles.
3. Sit by the child's bed with gradually decreasing pressure until they can sleep alone.
4. Alternatively, CIO (Cry It Out) method may work in 1-2 nights.

Sleep Training a 3-Year-Old (Parents' Role)

1. Establish a consistent bedtime routine.
2. Clearly communicate the expectation of staying in bed.
3. Introduce incentives like the "good sleeper fairy" or a call from a favorite character.
4. Be prepared for the child to test boundaries and consistently enforce the bedtime rule.

Note: In all cases, consistency, clear communication, and gradual adjustments are essential for successful sleep training. Parents must stay committed to the chosen method to achieve positive results.

17.7 Ready for Bed: Tips for Nighttime

Signs of an Overtired Baby

The baby may become cranky, very irritable, and cry uncontrollably. Other signs include looking away, staring at a wall (gaze aversion), eyes not moving around, yawning, slowing down of activity, slower sucking, quieter or calmer than typical, and drooping eyelids.

Tips for Nighttime Care

- Do not wake a sleeping baby at night, unless premature or as per Pediatrician's orders.
- Keep lights off or use a night light/red light when tending to the baby.
- Wait until the baby is at a full cry before attending to them.
- Avoid talking, eye contact, singing, rocking, and lights at night.
- Change and re-swaddle the baby first if needed. Feed only when necessary, using techniques to encourage eating.
- Burp the baby during the bottle-feeding process, ensuring to burp when there's less than an ounce left.
- Hold baby upright for 15-20 minutes to help the milk settle and prevent reflux.
- If the baby is wide awake when laid down, darken the room and leave. Allow the baby to self-soothe. Use pacifier or patting if needed.
- Cluster feed for the last two feeds if putting the baby down at 7 pm.

Hints for Newborn Care Specialists

- Swaddle tightly for nighttime and naps.
- Put them down for naps and bedtime awake but sleepy. Follow a consistent routine for both bedtime and naps.
- Establish a base for sleep patterns. Once a baby has slept for an equal amount of extended time (over three hours) for three nights in a row, he has established a new base. For example, if he slept for five hours in a row for three nights after sleeping only three hours as a norm, he has set a new base for himself. If on the fourth night he decides to wake up at four hours instead of the normal five, you should not feed him. You may give him a pacifier or just let him fuss. You can try to soothe him for the next hour, but try to keep him as close to that five hour mark as possible. You may find it beneficial to move at 30 minute increments rather than 60 minute.
- Use the pacifier strategically to soothe but avoid creating habits. Hold the pacifier in the baby's mouth until they go back to sleep. Once they are in deep sleep, remove the pacifier.
- Avoid starting habits you don't want to continue, like sleeping in different places or excessive rocking. Remember that anything done consecutively for three *times* (not days) becomes a habit to a baby.

- Have quality awake time each day, with one session between 4 pm and 7 pm or two hours before bedtime.
- Feed every three hours during the day, doing a full feed each time.
- Gradually lengthen awake time every three days, avoiding overstimulation.

17.8 Feeding for Sleep Training

For a baby sleeping through the night, the recommended feeding amount during the day is calculated as 2 ½ times their body weight (in pounds) divided by the number of feeds per day until they start solids. This formula serves as a general guide.

If the baby is fussy and inconsolable within one hour of the last feeding, you may attempt to feed more. Beyond one hour since the last feeding, wait until the next scheduled feeding.

It should take approximately 20 minutes to feed the baby using a bottle.

17.9 Newborn Naps

Scheduling is crucial for napping, both for newborns and older babies. A good 3-hour schedule is essential for newborns, involving 1 ¼ - 1 ½ hours of awake time followed by swaddling and putting them down. Up to approximately six months old, babies will continue with a morning and afternoon nap, taking a quick 30 - 45 minute catnap late in the afternoon.

17.10 Sleep Training for Multiple Babies

Consistency and repetition are crucial to working with multiples. Our goal will be to get the babies on the same schedule.

When you have more than one baby, you use the same methods to teach them to sleep as you would with just one baby. However, it can be more complicated if one baby wakes the other. If this happens, you should separate the babies into different rooms or at least different cribs and train them to sleep individually. Watch which one wakes up first, and keep track of this information. Let the baby who sleeps longer continue doing so, gradually adjusting the other baby's routine until they are both on the same schedule.

Chapter 18: Baby's Health and Wellness

18.1 Infant Poop Guide

An infant's poop can be a range of different consistencies and colors during their first few months of life. While this is normal, it is important to learn how to recognize unhealthy baby poop and to know what to do if it happens.

Your baby's first poops will be dark green/black and have a tar-like consistency. This poop is called meconium, and it is made up of cells, protein, fats, amniotic fluid, and intestinal secretions such as bile. Babies typically pass meconium in the first few hours and days after birth. This poop is sometimes hard to clean; the best way to clean is with coconut oil or olive oil on a clean cloth or wipe.

A bowel movement must occur before the baby is ready to leave the hospital. After that, it is typical for a bowel movement to happen with every diaper change in the first couple of days after birth. Newborns poop frequently, sometimes after every feed. Infants older than three weeks may poop from eight to twelve times a day to less than once a day.

Breast milk and formula can also influence the color of the baby's stool. In breastfed babies, the stool is yellowish and can change color according to what the mother is eating. Bottle-fed babies' stools are generally more uniform in color and consistency. Colors range anywhere from yellow to greenish-brown. However, red or white poop often signals health issues that require medical attention. Black stool from babies older than one week may also cause concern.

Healthy poop can be shades of yellow, orange, brown, or green, and the texture may be runny to reasonably firm. It should not be hard or watery.

If the baby is experiencing a cold, the diaper may have mucus instead of poop. Talk to the pediatrician if the baby doesn't have a cold and the diaper has mucus.

18.2 Health Warning Signs in Newborn Infants

As a new parent or caregiver of a newborn, it's crucial to recognize warning signs that may indicate a health problem or emergency. Here are common warning signs in newborns:

- **Difficulty Breathing:** Rapid breathing over 60 per minute, noisy breathing, grunting or whistling sounds, extra breathing effort, or bluish skin may indicate a respiratory problem.
- **High Fever:** Fever in a newborn, 100.4 degrees or higher, especially when accompanied by lethargy, poor feeding, or vomiting, could signal an infection.
- **Jaundice:** Yellow skin and yellow whites of the eyes suggest jaundice, indicating a potential issue with the baby's liver.
- **Poor Feeding:** If the baby isn't feeding well or lacks appetite, it could point to a digestive problem or infection.
- **Excessive Crying:** Unsoothable excessive crying might indicate pain, discomfort, or illness.
- **Lethargy:** Overly sleepy or difficult-to-wake behavior could indicate a severe condition like sepsis or meningitis.
- **Unusual Skin Changes:** Rashes, blisters, or other skin changes may signify infection, allergic reactions, or health problems.
- **Abnormal Body Movements:** Seizures, tremors, or jerking could be signs of a neurological condition.

In addition to these, watch for specific concerns within the first few days at home:

- No urine in the first 24 hours.
- No bowel movement in the first 48 hours.
- Rectal temperature over 100.4°F (38°C) or less than 97.5°F (36.5°C).
- Pulling in of the ribs with respiration.
- Weak cry or whimper.
- Any missing reflexes; inform the mother if any are noticed.

Seek immediate medical attention if you observe any warning signs or other symptoms. Don't hesitate to have the parents call the doctor or go to the emergency room if there are concerns about the baby's health.

18.3 Infant Ailments

Infants are vulnerable to various ailments due to their underdeveloped immune systems. Here are some common and uncommon ailments that infants may experience.

Common Ailments

- **Common Cold:** Infants can catch colds easily due to their underdeveloped immune systems. The symptoms include cough, runny nose, and fever.
- **Ear Infection:** This is a common ailment in infants, which bacterial or viral infections can cause. The symptoms include ear pain, fever, and irritability.
- **Gastroenteritis** is an inflammation of the digestive tract that causes vomiting and diarrhea.
- **Teething:** Teething is a natural process where a baby's teeth begin to emerge from the gums, causing discomfort and irritability.

Uncommon Ailments

- **Bronchiolitis:** An infection that causes inflammation of the small airways in the lungs; the symptoms include coughing, wheezing, and difficulty breathing.
- **Pertussis:** A bacterial infection that causes severe coughing spells, making it difficult for infants to breathe.
- **Meningitis:** An infection of the protective membranes surrounding the brain and spinal cord. The symptoms include fever, headache, and neck stiffness.
- **Kawasaki Disease:** A rare condition that causes inflammation of blood vessels throughout the body; the symptoms include fever, rash, and swollen lymph nodes.

It is essential to seek medical attention if the infant shows any symptoms of illness. Early diagnosis and treatment can prevent the condition from becoming severe.

18.4 Reflux

Reflux, where the stomach contents flow back into the esophagus, is common in newborns. In severe cases, this is sometimes referred to as gastroesophageal reflux (GER) or gastroesophageal reflux disease (GERD).

Newborns are more likely to experience reflux due to their lower esophageal sphincter (LES), a muscle that prevents stomach contents from flowing back into the esophagus, not being fully developed. Additionally, the position of a newborn's stomach, which is high up in the abdomen, may make it easier for the contents to flow back up.

For some babies, reflux is accompanied by mucus. What is happening is the acid in their digestive system irritates the esophagus, causing a burning sensation. The body responds by producing excessive phlegm to try and coat the irritated tissue. There may also be chronic ear infections and bad breath or sour breath. The child may have excessive gas or wheezing or make gargling sounds. "Failure to thrive" with a lack of weight gain or excessive weight gain may also indicate reflux.

Another possible reflux cause is artificial DHA/AHA added to formulas and prenatal vitamins.

Many parents overfeed the baby, thinking the baby is hungry when it is just trying to soothe reflux symptoms. A pacifier is more appropriate in this situation.

Symptoms that may indicate reflux:

- Spitting up and vomiting
- Projectile vomiting
- Hard hiccups
- Discomfort when lying on the back
- Crying and pulling away from the bottle or breast while feeding
- Gulping with painful swallowing
- Chronic cough or congestion, worse while lying down (not related to a cold)
- Waking suddenly with a painful cry
- Hoarseness
- Arching the back when drinking or while lying down
- Frequent choking or gagging episodes
- Small feeds
- Frequent feeds to comfort or chase the burn
- Sour face while swallowing
- Chronic irritability
- Strong need to suck, especially after being fed
- Wheezing or gurgling sounds
- Excessive gas, hard belly
- Only happy when held
- Excessive colic

- Frequent colds or ear infections
- Displaying a fear of food or unwillingness to eat
- Feeding only when drowsy
- Large number of wet diapers due to frequent feeding
- Difficulty settling
- Frequent waking in the night
- Prefers to be upright versus lying down
- Recurrent ear, throat, sinus, or chest infections or croup
- Excessive salivation
- Behavioural issues
- Sticking their hand/fingers/fist down throat

Silent Reflux

Silent reflux in infants is not as apparent because there is no spitting up, making it harder to detect. For some babies, the reflux does not reach their mouth; it may come halfway up and back down, causing a lot of burning and discomfort. It may also come through the nose. The main symptom in these cases is constant "comfort nursing" or a continuous need to suck. These babies are often overfed, which makes the reflux worse.

In addition to the symptoms above, a baby with silent reflux may also have the following:

- Poor or rapid weight gain
- Painful wake-ups from sleep or poor sleeping habits
- Demands to be carried constantly
- Red or salmon-colored throat
- Blood in the stool or spit-up (see pediatrician if blood in the stool)

Reflux and Nursing

Doctors sometimes suggest that mothers don't breastfeed babies with reflux. However, we don't recommend avoiding breastfeeding. If you notice reflux symptoms, we suggest moms start pumping to maintain their milk supply. Also, reconsider the mom's diet by eliminating acidic foods like tomatoes, onions, chocolate, peppers, fried food, milk, and dairy products. Gradually reintroduce them individually, and keep track of how the baby reacts. Permanently eliminate foods that cause issues.

Cow's milk protein sensitivity or allergy can contribute to reflux. To check if the breastfed baby is sensitive, the mother should avoid all cow's milk protein forms for two weeks (including milk, yogurt, ice cream, cheese, butter, casein, and whey). If the baby improves, the mother should continue avoiding all dairy products. Some mothers can tolerate small amounts of dairy, while others should avoid it altogether. Explore non-dairy sources of calcium if needed.

Potential Triggers for Reflux

- Teething
- Crawling
- Illness
- Vaccinations
- Constipation
- Overly tired or out of routine

Reflux Remedies

- Feed baby in an upright or sitting position
- Avoid moving the baby a lot after the feed; placing the baby in a bouncy seat for 30 minutes after feeding is best
- Avoid laying the baby flat right after feeding
- Swaddling can be calming when baby has reflux
- Swinging and vibration are very soothing
- Allow the baby to use a pacifier to self-soothe between feeds
- Allow baby to sleep on their tummy when they are being supervised and never left alone in this position
- Use Colic Calm (a homeopathic remedy) or a gentle form of activated charcoal several times a day
- Consider organic, liquid formula
- Consider pea formula or hypo-allergenic formula
- Probiotics may be helpful.
- We don't recommend avoiding breastfeeding. If reflux symptoms are noticed, pumping may be helpful in maintaining milk supply. The mother's diet may need to be closely examined. Eliminate acidic foods.
- Allow baby to sleep on their tummy when they are being closely supervised and never left along in that position.

Possible Natural Remedies to Try

Chamomile: Chamomile has anti-inflammatory and anti-spasmodic properties that can help soothe the digestive tract and reduce acid reflux symptoms in babies. You can give the baby chamomile tea alone or mixed with breast milk or formula. Make sure the tea is lukewarm and not too hot.

Fennel: Fennel is another herb that can help ease digestive discomfort and reduce acid reflux symptoms in babies. You can make fennel tea by steeping a teaspoon of fennel seeds in a cup of hot water for 10 minutes. After the tea has cooled, give the baby a teaspoon mixed with breast milk or formula.

Baking soda in warm water: If the baby will drink it, add a teaspoon of baking soda to a half-cup of warm water. The baking soda neutralizes the stomach acid.

18.5 Colic

Colic is a common condition that affects some newborns and infants up to 4-5 months old, starting any time after three weeks. It is characterized by periods of intense crying and fussiness when the baby seems inconsolable for no apparent reason. It typically occurs in the late afternoon or evening and lasts several hours. One measure of whether it is colic is the rule of threes: the crying lasts more than three hours a day, more than three days a week, for more than three weeks. The exact cause of colic is unknown, but it is thought to be related to digestive issues, such as gas or indigestion, a developing nervous system, maternal anxiety, or brain immaturity.

The symptoms of colic can include:

- Crying that is high-pitched, continuous, and inconsolable.
- Pulling up the legs to the abdomen.
- Clenched fists.
- A flushed face.

The baby may also have trouble sleeping or eating.

Troubleshooting Colic

Make sure the baby isn't overstimulated. Overstimulation can cause the baby to cry inconsolably. Attempts to calm them with rocking, singing, or walking may worsen the situation.

The child's biological schedule can be disrupted if you miss the baby's bedtime or feeding times. A baby will sleep better, longer, and deeper when kept to a routine schedule.

Some babies struggle to transition from wakefulness to sleep, leading to increased crying in the evening. Swaddle the baby, put them down fed, dry, and if possible, awake.

Remedies for Colic

There are several strategies that parents can try to help soothe a colicky baby, including:

- Holding the baby in a vertical position during and after feeding to help reduce gas.
- Using a pacifier to help soothe the baby.
- Swaddling the baby.
- Providing gentle motion, such as rocking or bouncing, to help calm the baby.
- Playing white noise or other calming sounds to help the baby relax.

The Bicycle Exercise to Help Relieve Gas

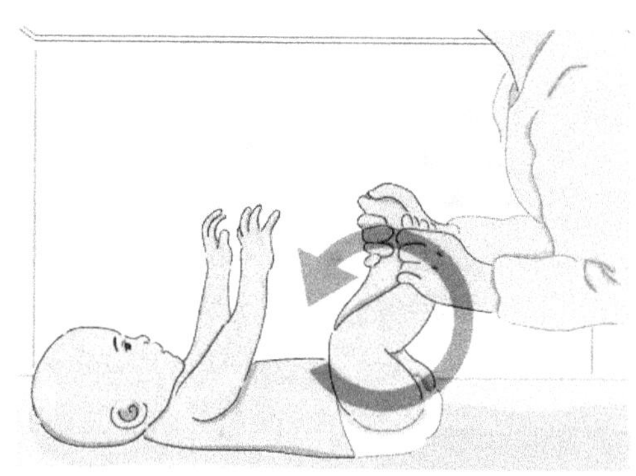

If the baby is lying on their back, gently move their legs back and forth to imitate riding a bicycle. This exercise helps with intestinal motion and can expel trapped gas. You can also bend their legs and gently push their knees toward their tummy.

Massage to Relieve Gas

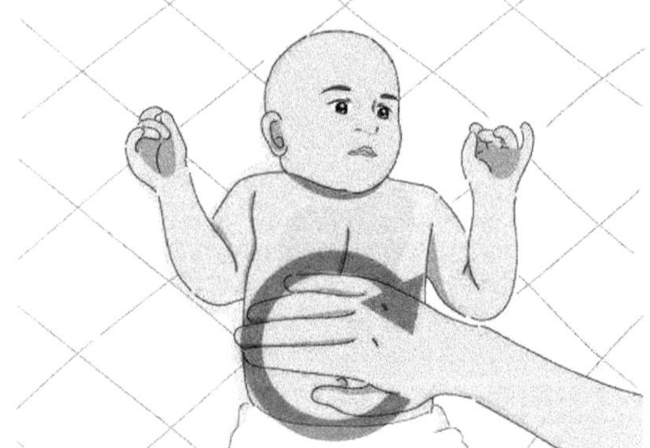

Baby massage is a method nurses use to soothe infants with gas bubbles. Lie the baby down on their back, then start rubbing their tummy in a clockwise circular motion. By doing this across the baby's tummy in a smooth, gentle motion, you're triggering activity in their abdomen that can help them pass those trapped gas bubbles.

Parents or caregivers need to remain patient and seek support when dealing with a colicky baby, as it can be a challenging and exhausting experience. Parents should also consult with a pediatrician to rule out any underlying medical conditions and to discuss treatment options, if necessary.

18.6 Thrush in Infants

Thrush is a common fungal infection caused by an overgrowth of the fungus Candida Albicans. Symptoms of thrush in infants may include:

- White or yellow patches in the mouth, tongue, lips, or gums.

- Irritability or fussiness during feeding or sucking.
- Refusing to feed or difficulty in feeding.
- Soreness or redness in the mouth.

Thrush can be treated with antifungal medications prescribed by a doctor. In addition to medication, do the following to help prevent the spread of thrush:

- Boiling or sterilizing pacifiers, bottle nipples, and other feeding equipment.
- Wiping the inside of the baby's mouth with a clean, damp cloth after each feeding.
- Avoid sharing towels or other items that come into contact with the baby's mouth.
- It is important to seek medical attention if you suspect the baby has thrush, as it can be uncomfortable and may interfere with feeding.

18.7 Cradle Cap

When a rash shows up on the scalp, it is likely cradle cap. It might start with scaling and redness on the scalp but can also appear in other areas. Cradle cap looks like greasy, yellow, scaly patches on the scalp skin. This happens when there are a lot of oil-producing sebaceous glands.

Cradle cap is a common skin condition in infants, starting in the first weeks of life and gradually fading in a few weeks or months. It's usually not uncomfortable or itchy and is not harmful.

The exact cause of this rash is unknown, but it may be influenced by hormonal changes during pregnancy, which stimulate oil glands.

Treatment of Cradle Cap

If the baby only has cradle cap on the scalp, you can treat it at home. Wash the hair more often with a mild baby shampoo and gently brush to remove scales. Some parents use olive oil or coconut oil; rub it on the scales, leave it overnight (cover the baby's head), then shampoo and brush it out in the morning. You can also apply olive oil or coconut oil to the scalp, rub it around, and wash away the scales.

Medicated shampoos with sulfur and 2 percent salicylic acid may work faster but irritate. Use them only after talking to a pediatrician. The doctor might prescribe additional medication for the scales and redness.

If regular shampooing doesn't help or the rash spreads, especially to the face and neck, consult a pediatrician. They might suggest a stronger shampoo and prescribe a cortisone cream or lotion. One percent hydrocortisone cream is commonly used.

Preventing Cradle Cap

After improvement, you can usually prevent cradle cap from coming back by using olive oil or coconut oil. Occasionally, a stronger medicated shampoo may be needed, but let your pediatrician decide. After the child's first birthday, cradle cap generally doesn't return until puberty.

18.8 Shaken Baby Syndrome

Shaken Baby Syndrome is a severe brain injury that happens when a baby or child up to five years old is shaken violently, causing the brain to hit against the skull. Because babies have large heads and weak neck muscles, their brains can easily bounce inside the skull. This can lead to bruising, swelling, and bleeding of the brain, sometimes causing permanent, severe brain injury or even death. Other injuries can include:

- Bleeding in the retinas.
- Damage to the spinal cord and neck.
- Fractures of the ribs and bones.

Often, there are no obvious outward signs of this kind of injury.

The symptoms of Shaken Baby Syndrome may not show up immediately, but they can include extreme irritability, lethargy, difficulty feeding, breathing problems, convulsions, vomiting, and pale or bluish skin. Shaken Baby Syndrome usually happens due to child abuse and not during regular play. It often occurs when a baby cries for a long time, perhaps due to illness or colic. In most cases, the person responsible is the father, followed by the mother, and then a caregiver.

It's crucial to remember: NEVER shake a baby. Half of the babies who are shaken die. If you feel like you're losing control, put the baby down and step away. Shower, go outside, or do something to distract yourself from frustration. Babies with colic are at the highest risk, as they can cry inconsolably for a whole day. It's challenging, and it's okay to feel frustrated. Don't blame yourself; take a break, have a tea, relax, and return to the situation.

Injuries from shaking a baby can include learning disabilities, partial or total blindness, death, delays in development, spinal injury, speech problems, paralysis, hearing loss, impaired use of arms and legs, mental retardation, and brain damage with seizures.

18.9 Positional Plagiocephaly

A baby's head bones are very thin and flexible, making the head soft and easy to shape. In the first few months, babies can't roll over on their own because they're not strong enough. If a baby often looks in one direction or lies on their back often, part of the skull may become flat. This flattening is called Positional Plagiocephaly, and it is due to constant pressure on one part of the skull. This issue is noticed around 2 or 3 months of age when a flattened area, a bulging forehead, and a pushed-forward ear can be observed.

Positional Plagiocephaly happens when a baby spends a lot of time lying on their back. Even though this is the case, it's still recommended to let babies sleep on their backs to reduce the risk of Sudden Infant Death Syndrome (SIDS). Another cause might be Torticallis or underdeveloped neck muscles, which can be too tight or uneven, making the head turn naturally in one direction.

In multiple births, babies may be born with Plagiocephaly if they are pressed onto the mother's pelvic bone or another sibling in the uterus for long periods.

What does it look like?

A baby with Positional Plagiocephaly has a flat area on the back of the skull, which can be uneven if the baby prefers resting on one side. Sometimes, it can be symmetric if the baby always lies in the middle of the back of the head.

Treatment

- When putting the baby down to sleep, alternate the head's position each time.
- Change the crib's position so the baby can look at different things.
- Use tummy time when the baby is awake and you are in the room.
- Avoid extended time in the car seat, bouncer, or other flat or hard inclined surfaces. If these are necessary, you can use rice socks or rolled up burp cloths or blankets to position baby to be off the affected flat side while in these seats.
- If there's no improvement within 2 or 3 months, consult a pediatric surgeon.
- Most problems resolve once the baby begins to roll over and move their head independently. It's important to note Plagiocephaly doesn't affect a child's brain growth or cause developmental delays or brain damage.

18.10 Jaundice

Jaundice happens in about 50% of full-term babies and about 75% of premature babies. When a baby has jaundice, their skin and the whites of their eyes turn yellow. It often starts in the face and can spread to the rest of the body, even making the fingernails look yellow. Some babies with jaundice might sleep a lot and not eat well.

Jaundice, also called hyperbilirubinemia, is when there's too much bilirubin in the blood. In the womb, babies need extra blood cells for oxygen, and after birth, these cells break down, releasing bilirubin into the blood. The baby's liver is supposed to remove bilirubin, but sometimes it can't because the liver is still developing. Babies usually get rid of bilirubin through bowel movements, so the more a baby eats and has bowel movements, the faster the bilirubin leaves their system. If the baby's eating is restricted or scheduled, and bowel movements are infrequent, bilirubin can be absorbed back into the system, causing the yellowing of the skin and eyes. If jaundice is suspected, the pediatrician will check the bilirubin level in the baby's system.

There are four types of jaundice in infants:

- **Pathological Jaundice:** Requires immediate medical attention. Occurs 24 hours after birth due to liver disease or blood incompatibility. Signs include a fast rise in bilirubin, yellow skin and eyes, sleepiness, and poor feeding.
- **Physiological Jaundice:** Appears around the third day and disappears within 10-12 days. It's common in breastfed and bottle-fed babies. While some doctors may not treat it, others might use phototherapy (indirect sunlight) or suggest supplementing formulas.
- **Breastfeeding Jaundice:** Occurs when babies haven't been fed enough. It happens 3-5 days after birth. Signs include yellow skin and eyes, sleepiness, poor eating, weight loss, and fewer than four bowel movements daily. Feeding every three hours during the day can help prevent it.
- **Breast Milk Jaundice:** This can happen in up to 30% of newborns. The cause is unknown. It appears 4-6 days after birth, peaking 10-14 days after. It might stay elevated for months. Some substances in breast milk may affect the baby's liver. The doctor might suggest stopping breastfeeding, although it hasn't been proven harmful. Signs include yellow skin and eyes, an alert and active baby, weight gain, frequent feeding, and more than four bowel movements.

18.11 Sudden Infant Death Syndrome (SIDS)

Researchers are finding a connection between sudden infant death and problems in the unconscious part of the brain. A study suggests that babies who die of Sudden Infant Death Syndrome (SIDS) might struggle with producing Serotonin, a brain chemical that helps control the heart and breathing without conscious effort. According to a team from Harvard Medical School and the Children's Hospital in Boston, this might explain why some babies who sleep on their stomachs or have reduced oxygen during sleep struggle to wake up.

Risk Factors of SIDS

- Parent or caregiver smoking.
- Sleeping on the tummy.
- Premature birth or very low birth weight.
- Overheating during sleep.
- Sleeping on a soft surface.
- Mother using drugs during pregnancy.
- Mother under 20 during pregnancy.
- Experiencing an apparent life-threatening event.
- African American infants have 2.5 times higher SIDS risk than white infants and Native American babies have three times the risk.
- Boys are more likely to die of SIDS than girls.

How to Reduce SIDS Risk

- Put a baby to sleep on its back.
- Take care of the mom's health during pregnancy.
- Avoid smoking around the baby.
- Choose bedding carefully.
- Prevent overheating.
- Reduce exposure to infection.

Despite clinical details, SIDS can't be predicted or detected beforehand. It happens suddenly and is not related to a sick child. Some monitoring devices like the V-Sense Baby Monitor can provide extra peace of mind by sounding an alarm if there's no movement or breathing for a specific time.

18.12 Respiratory Syncytial Virus (RSV)

Respiratory Syncytial Virus (RSV) is a common respiratory infection that can lead to a severe cold or pneumonia in babies and young kids. According to the Centers for Disease Control and Prevention (CDC), almost all children in the United States get infected with RSV by the age of three.

RSV results in about 90,000 hospitalizations and 4,500 deaths annually.

For most cases, RSV shows up as a mild cold. But for children under six months, premature babies, or those with heart defects or chronic lung diseases, the risk of hospitalization is up to six times higher.

RSV spreads like a cold through coughing, sneezing, or contact with contaminated surfaces. If you have a cold and care for an infant, washing your hands after blowing your nose, coughing, or sneezing is crucial. RSV is most contagious during the first two to four days but can spread up to three weeks after the infection starts. It occurs throughout the year but peaks in late fall to early spring, especially in January and February.

Symptoms of RSV are similar to a common cold, including a runny nose, cough, sore throat, and mild fever. Symptoms may involve high fever, severe cough, wheezing, and rapid or difficult breathing in young children and infants. If these symptoms occur, calling a pediatrician right away is recommended.

No specific treatment is needed for mild cases except for managing symptoms, such as using a humidifier, encouraging fluid intake, using saline drops for the nose, and giving acetaminophen to reduce fever. Severe cases may require hospital treatment. Most children recover in one to two weeks.

Preventing RSV involves frequent handwashing, cleaning toys, and not sharing cups and utensils. To protect infants from RSV, keep them away from people with cold symptoms.

Two medicines are approved to prevent severe RSV infections in high-risk infants, like those born prematurely or with chronic lung disease. These medicines are given in five monthly doses during RSV/flu season.

18.13 Projectile Vomiting

Projectile vomiting is when a baby forcefully throws up, like spraying milk across the room. It's normal if it happens once or twice daily due to overfeeding, underburping, or jostling the baby too much. It becomes a concern if it persists, leading to weight loss, failure to gain weight, signs of dehydration, or a swollen stomach after feeding. Your doctor may check for Pyloric Stenosis, a condition where a muscle at the stomach's end blocks food from entering the intestines, causing projectile vomiting. Surgery can fix this, and recovery is quick.

18.14 Colds

Infants will have occasional breathing issues as their lungs and immune system develop. If a baby catches a cold, this section suggests actions to take.

Vaporizer

To help a congested baby breathe better:

1. Consider using a vaporizer.
2. Choose a hot mist vaporizer over a cool mist one, as specialists favor it for killing bacteria and mold.
3. Clean it weekly with a bleach solution, change the water daily, and use only distilled water.
4. Keep it about two feet away from the baby and aim the mist at their nose. You can add Eucalyptus to optimize its effect.

If you don't have a vaporizer, you can use the steam from a shower in the bathroom to break up congestion. Never put the baby in the shower; instead, sit with them on the toilet. If a cold lasts more than five days without improvement, consult a doctor.

For nasal discharge, clear mucus is normal during a cold or teething. Yellow or green, thick discharge with a fever indicates an infection. If it persists, consult a doctor. If there's eye discharge, see a doctor if it doesn't improve.

To use a nasal aspirator for congestion:

1. Make a saline solution with a pinch of salt in warm distilled water.
2. Drop a few solution drops into each nostril.
3. Let it sit for a few seconds to loosen mucus.
4. Use the nasal aspirator by squeezing the bulb, placing it in one nostril, and releasing it to suck up mucus. Repeat on the other side.
5. Between uses, squeeze out the mucus onto a tissue.
6. Wash the aspirator with soap and hot water after each use. Avoid making this a daily practice to protect the baby's delicate nose tissues. Use it only in cases of congestion.

18.15 Infant Failure to Thrive

Infant Failure to Thrive (FTT) is when an infant or young child is not gaining weight, growing, or developing at the expected rate for age and gender. The condition is typically diagnosed when a child's weight or height is below the third percentile or has dropped two significant percentiles quickly. FFT happens in about 5-10% of babies, mostly in premature cases.

There are many causes of FTT, the most common of which is malnutrition, either as an organic problem or an energy imbalance. Malnutrition results from the following:

- inadequate caloric intake
- feeding difficulties
- food allergies or intolerances
- malabsorption
- digestive or metabolic disorders such as celiac disease, cystic fibrosis, or liver disease
- excessive caloric expenditure.
- hyperthyroidism
- chronic infections
- other chronic illnesses

FTT can also be impacted by:

- Premature birth, especially with growth issues
- Maternal smoking, alcohol, or drug use during pregnancy
- Mechanical problems like cleft lip or palate
- Poor feeding skills by the caregiver
- Dysfunctional family interactions
- Difficult parent-child interactions
- Lack of social support
- Lack of parenting preparation
- Emotional deprivation
- Hyper-vigilance (always on guard or tense)

While we can't fix a dysfunctional family, we can help with parenting prep and emotional support. We need to identify issues early and guide parents. Social support is crucial; we can connect families with local help.

Failure to Thrive Symptoms

FTT babies struggle to gain weight properly. An average newborn gains about half a pound per week. Some variation is okay, but losing or barely gaining weight is a concern. Babies should regain birth weight within two weeks, double it in 6 months, and triple it in 12 months.

Other symptoms to look for:

- Edema (water retention)
- Rashes
- Changes in hair or skin
- Maternal detachment

Inorganic causes, like postpartum depression in the mother, can affect a baby's emotional development. Babies sense their mother's emotions, so a stressed or angry mom can impact the baby negatively. It's vital to be aware of these factors and offer support when needed.

It is essential to address the underlying cause of FTT as early as possible. Treatment may involve addressing feeding difficulties, modifying the diet, or using nutritional supplements. In some cases, hospitalization may be necessary to manage severe cases of FTT. A healthcare provider should be consulted for concerns about a child's growth or development.

18.16 Chemicals in Baby Products

The world is being bombarded by chemicals in the products we use. Babies are the most vulnerable to these effects. Never assume that a brand-name manufacturer won't include dangerous substances in their baby items. To be safe, you must conduct your own study.

You can find out what chemicals are in your products and those you use on infants by visiting http://www.ewg.org/skindeep/. Here are a few to watch out for:

- **Propylene Glycol (Antifreeze):** Found in lotions and soap, this chemical alters skin structure, allowing other chemicals to penetrate deeper into the skin, increasing the amounts reaching the bloodstream. It's been linked with skin conditions such as eczema and dermatitis. It's also found in some vitamins, foods, and toothpaste. Industrially, it's also found in antifreeze.
- **Sodium Lauryl Sulfate (SLS) or Sodium Laureth Sulfate (SLES):** Research shows that SLS and SLES may cause potentially carcinogenic nitrates and dioxins to form in shampoo and cleanser when bottles react with commonly used ingredients. Large amounts of nitrates may enter the bloodstream from just one shampooing. They can cause eye irritations, skin rashes, hair loss, scalp scurf (like dandruff), and allergic reactions. Industrial uses of SLS include engine degreasers and car wash soaps.
- SLS is also rapidly taken up and accumulated in eye tissue and is retained for up to five days. It denatures eye tissue proteins, permanently impairing development, and extends the healing time of the cornea surface for ten days (two days on average). Finally, tissues of young eyes may be more susceptible to alteration by SLS. SLS is found in almost

all toothpaste, shampoos, and bubble baths. Take a look at your toothpaste. Did you ever wonder why it says, "Keep out of the reach of children...if swallowed, contact a POISON CONTROL CENTER IMMEDIATELY?"

- **Methylparaben and propylparaben** may affect hormone levels, raise the risk of some cancers, impair fertility, or change a fetus's or young child's development. Numerous shampoos, lotions, and cosmetic products contain paraben as a common ingredient. Any ingredient name with the word "paraben" at the end could be highly hazardous.
- Another hazardous chemical is **diethanolamine**. It can be found in shampoos, conditioners, bubble baths, lotions, soaps, cosmetics, dishwashing, and laundry detergents.
- Disposable diapers consist of super-absorbent chemicals, paper pulps, and plastics. In a study from 1999, it was found that chemicals released by disposable diapers might contribute to or worsen asthma. Diapers were tested right after being removed from the packet, and the emissions were high enough to trigger breathing difficulties.
- Mylicon is often recommended for colic and gas by pediatricians. However, it contains, among other things, D&C Red 22, D&C Red 28, and many non-natural ingredients. We recommend a more natural product.
- Making anti-fungal baby wipes that are excellent for a baby's skin is possible without using chemicals or alcohol.
- Many ailments in a baby's life may be treated naturally without using drugs or chemicals. Products found on kitchen shelves can be used to treat diaper rash, cradle cap, and colic. Homeopathic and herbal treatments are entirely safe and highly effective, with no adverse side effects.

Endocrine Disruptors

The endocrine system is a network of glands, hormones, and receptors controlling bodily functions. It manages mood, growth, development, tissue function, sexual function, and reproduction.

In 1996, the Food Quality Protection Act was created to check contaminants for potential harm to the endocrine system. More than two decades later, the market is filled with chemicals that can impact your health, especially when combined in untested ways.

An endocrine disruptor can change the endocrine system's function, affecting your health or an unborn child. Chemicals that are endocrine disruptors may:

- Imitate hormones by binding to cellular receptors, causing responses at the wrong time

- Bind to receptors without activating them, preventing natural hormone binding
- Bind to blood transport proteins, altering natural hormone levels.
- Interfere with metabolic processes, affecting hormone synthesis or breakdown.

Chemicals to avoid are widespread. Check the bathroom for cosmetics, lotions, baby products, soaps, cleaning fluids, and deodorants. Avoid these twelve potential endocrine disruptors:

- Bisphenol A (BPA): Common in plastics, including reusable water bottles and resins lining some food cans and dental sealants. It can alter fetal development, increasing the risk of breast cancer.
- Bovine growth hormones: Added to commercial dairy, implicated as contributing to premature adolescence.
- Fluoride: In the U.S., fluoride in the water supply is linked to lower fertility rates, hormone disruption, and low sperm counts.
- Methoxychlor and Vinclozin: An insecticide and a fungicide that can cause changes in male mice born for as many as four subsequent generations after initial exposure.
- MSG: A neurotoxin and food additive linked to reduced fertility.
- Nonylphenol ethoxylates (NPEs): Potent endocrine disrupters in various products that mimic female hormones and affect gene expression and glandular system function. This is implicated in some marine species switching from male to female.
- Perfluorooctanoic acid (PFOA): Found in grease- and water-resistant coatings like Teflon and Gore-Tex. A likely carcinogen.
- Phthalates: Found in vinyl flooring, detergents, automotive plastics, soap, shampoo, deodorants, fragrances, hair spray, nail polish, plastic bags, food packaging, garden hoses, inflatable toys, blood-storage bags, and intravenous medical tubing. Exposure can lead to incomplete testicular descent in fetuses.
- Soy products: Loaded with hormone-like substances.
- Synthetically produced pharmaceuticals: Intended to be highly hormonally active, such as contraceptive pills and treatments for hormone-responsive cancers. Prolonged exposure increases the risk of severe chronic illness.
- Other natural chemicals: Toxins produced by plant components (phytoestrogens) and certain fungi.

- Other artificial chemicals and by-products released into the environment that include pesticides (pyrethroids, linuron, vinclozolin, fenitrothion, DDT, and other chlorinated compounds) and industrial chemicals (polychlorinated bisphenols - PCBs, and dioxins). These chemicals can affect a child's health, causing:
  - declining sperm counts
  - genital malformations
  - hormone-sensitive cancers
  - impaired neural development, memory problems
  - lower IQ
  - impaired sexual behavior
  - precocious puberty
  - delayed sexual development

18.17 How to Handle Infant Ailments

When you suspect the newborn is struggling with their health, the first step is to take the baby's temperature to check for a fever.

How to Take a Baby's Temperature

There are six ways to take a baby's temperature:

- **Rectal:** Taking a rectal temperature is the most accurate way to check for a fever. New thermometers have insertion guides and provide readings in 10 seconds.
  1. Shake the thermometer below 96°F.
  2. Apply lubricant to the tip.
  3. Lay the baby on their tummy on a firm surface.
  4. Insert the thermometer using the guide.
  5. Hold in place for the recommended time.
  6. Carefully slide out and read. Be aware the baby may poop.
- **Axillary:** Place the thermometer in the armpit.
  1. Press the baby's arm against their side.
  2. Remove after 4-5 minutes.
  3. An acceptable method; hospitals use; normal range is 95° - 99°F.

- **Oral:** Not recommended; pacifier thermometer works if needed.
- **Ear:** Suitable after six months.
  1. Lay baby on their back, pull the ear back, and point the thermometer into the ear canal.
  2. Activate and wait for the beep; use the highest reading.
  3. Normal range is 97.8° - 99.7°F.
- **Rolling Forehead Thermometer:** Effective when used correctly.
  1. Start at one temple and roll across the forehead and behind the ear.
  2. Must be precise for accuracy.
  3. Normal range is 95° - 99°F.
- **Forehead Strips:** Very inaccurate.

Fever Warning for Babies Under Three Months

- If the child is under three months old and has a fever for more than eight hours, call a healthcare professional.
- If the child seems lethargic, persistently vomits, is drowsy, not eating, and pale, call a healthcare professional immediately.
- Un-bundle the baby, increase fluids, and watch if the baby has a fever but doesn't seem very ill.

How to Lower a Temperature

A fever is the body's way to fight infection; in many cases, you can let it run its course. However, to alleviate the baby's discomfort, use the following to lower the temperature:

- Aspirin is not recommended for babies; use baby Tylenol. (Always use a Medicine Consent Form when administering any medication.)
- Encourage fluid intake.
- Keep the baby cool and not over-dressed.
- Give a lukewarm bath if the fever is 104°F or above; avoid cool baths.

When to Call the Doctor

- High fever for age
- Fever persists after a couple of days
- Constant crying or lethargy

- It's hard to wake up or limp
- Bulging soft spot
- Stiff neck or stomach pain
- Purple spots or rash
- Paleness or flushing
- Difficulty breathing

When Talking to the Doctor, Provide...

- When the fever started
- How fast it increased
- Fever pattern
- Baby's overall condition
- Other symptoms
- Parental concern
- Diarrhea frequency
- Number of wet diapers in 24 hours
- Baby's food intake in 24 hours

18.18 Administering Medications

Oral Medications

Use a syringe or dropper for drops. Avoid using a spoon.

- Slowly squirt the medication between the tongue and the side of the mouth. Let the baby swallow.
- Don't squirt the medication into the back of the baby's mouth; it triggers the gag reflex. Putting it directly on the tongue might make the baby push it out.
- The best way is to put it in the bottle nipple or use a medicine pacifier. The baby will likely take it without realizing it's medicine.
- Don't add medication to a full bottle; you won't know how much the baby gets. Inform your Pediatrician if the baby vomits or can't keep anything down; they might suggest a suppository.
- Don't double the dose if you miss one; give the missed dose as soon as possible and adjust the schedule accordingly.

Ear Drops

- Lay the child down and turn their head to one side.
- Gently pull the ear slightly down and back to create a direct route for the medication.

- Keep the baby lying on the side for a few minutes.

Eye Drops

1. Lay the child down and gently pull the lower lid down.
2. Apply the ointment or drops.

18.19 Natural and Safe Remedies

Suggestions for natural remedies and methods are listed in the section where they best apply.

Some cosmetic brands we found safe for babies, without chemicals, include Avalon, Burt's Bees, Aubrey's, Healthy Timez, and California Baby.

18.20 Newborn Safety

Most childhood accidents are preventable. Use common sense, prioritize safety, and never leave a child unattended. Here are additional tips for baby safety:

- When installing safety devices, consider your child's determination to explore. Test the item's durability to withstand your child's actions.
- Place a fire rescue decal in the baby's window for emergency guidance.
- Remove potential stepping stools or ladders if other children might attempt to climb into the crib.
- Use a net tent over the crib if there's a cat in the house or to protect against scorpions. It also prevents other children from throwing things into the crib while the baby sleeps.
- Reverse the lock on the bedroom door to avoid accidentally locking the baby inside.
- Secure cabinets, closets, or drawers where hazardous items are stored. Use door handle covers to keep toddlers out of restricted areas. Safety gates are helpful for stairs, open windows, kitchen, or bathroom entries. Wall-mounted gates provide additional security. Secure anything a baby can reach, climb to, under, or through.

18.21 The Effect of Electro Magnetic Fields (EMFs) on Infants

We're all used to modern technology and its convenience, but many are unaware of the possible health risks, to infants in particular, that come with these high-tech gadgets so prevalent in our world.

Computers, microwaves, cellphones, Wi-Fi routers, and other appliances produce invisible energy called electromagnetic field waves that may cause harm.

So, what is an EMF, and why should we be concerned?

Since the beginning of the solar system, the sun has sent out waves that create electric and magnetic fields known as radiation. The energy radiating out is visible light.

Mimicking the sun's energy, electric power lines and indoor lighting now criss-crossing the world also emit EMFs. Once scientists learned that the power grid was sending EMFs, it followed that many appliances that use electricity also cause EMFs, along with X-rays and some medical imagining procedures like MRIs.

While EMFs cannot damage DNA or cells directly, some scientists speculate that EMFs could cause cancer and other health problems by reducing melatonin hormone levels, which regulate sleep. Sleep is crucial for a healthy life. The new diagnosis of "EMF Hypersensitivity Syndrome" is seen more frequently, with one of the main symptoms being insomnia.

There are two types of EMF exposure:

- Non-Ionizing Radiation (Low-level Radiation): Mild and thought to be harmless to people. Appliances like microwave ovens, computers, cellphones, Bluetooth devices, power lines, wireless routers, MRIs, and house energy meters emit low-level radiation.
- Ionizing Radiation (High-level Radiation): Examples are ultraviolet light and X-rays.

Symptoms of EMF Exposure

The body's nervous system function and cell health can be affected by EMFs, while cancer and unusual growths may be symptoms of very high EMF exposure. Other symptoms may include sleep disturbances, depression, tiredness, headache, dizziness, anxiety, nausea, loss of appetite, weight loss, changes in memory, lack of concentration, skin burning and tingling, and changes in an electroencephalogram (which measures electrical activity in the brain).

The symptoms of EMF exposure are vague, and diagnosis from symptoms is difficult.

How EMF Radiation from Electronics Can Affect Children

Children's bodies are much different than adults on a physical, chemical, and biological level because children are still developing. As a result, EMF radiation can have a profound effect on their bodies.

Early studies show that EMF from cell phones can penetrate a child's brain much more than adults. This may be due to the higher water content in children's tissues. EMFs can do more damage over a larger area because cells split and grow as a child matures, which can develop into permanent biological effects like ADHD, autism, and obesity.

Educated caregivers and parents must realize that cell phones may harm infants because their bodies are still maturing, and the technology is still very new.

Protection from EMF Exposure

The data from different researchers provide conflicting results. Some studies show increased childhood leukemia and brain tumor rates, while others claim there is no link between cancer and EMF exposure. Since the evidence is inconsistent, more research is needed, especially on the long-term health effects of EMF exposure. Even a slight increase in cancer risk would be significant, considering how widespread exposure everyone gets in today's societies.

Since harmful effects from even environmental level exposure are possible, the public should follow the precautionary principle and limit exposure as much as possible.

Keeping a distance between the source of EMF and the body is the best way to diminish its effect. For example, don't charge the phone where the infant sleeps. You may also look into EMF protectors, which shield EMF and reduce exposure from electronic devices that emit electromagnetic waves. EMF protectors are especially recommended for babies and small children as they are the most vulnerable age group.

Chapter 19: Looking Out for Mother

We can help the mother, and as a result, the family, in five ways:

1. **First is emotional care.** When we arrive, we bring emotional stability and support to the mom. We connect, encourage, and empower her during this critical time after giving birth. We provide the emotional connection she needs to handle the changes.
2. **The second is information and resources.** We offer practical advice for situations the mom is facing, like a crying baby or breastfeeding concerns. We give information in a way that's easy to understand and provide resources like recommended pediatricians and lactation consultants.
3. **Third is physical care.** We offer hands-on support by showing practical solutions, like changing a diaper or positioning the baby safely. We empower parents by demonstrating these tasks and building their confidence.
4. **Fourth is advocacy.** We work alongside the mom, respecting her choices and preferences. We provide information and advice but ultimately let her make decisions, giving her the power to choose. Let the mom know we will always ask permission and follow their preference, even when we have a favorite way of doing something.
5. **Fifth is family care.** We help strengthen the family unit, offering guidance on connecting with siblings and creating harmony. We are mindful of different family dynamics. We always remember to include the father, as they sometimes feel powerless. We also teach dads practical methods; they need reassurance and empowerment as much as moms. Additionally, we should be open and sensitive to various family types, including LGBTQ families, visually impaired parents, those with different religious beliefs, and diverse cultural backgrounds.

We aim to make a safe environment when we enter the mom's space, her room, or home. She should feel comfortable being herself. We encourage her to return to her daily routine.

We also help parents establish a new routine with the baby. We show them practical ways to balance their daily life while prioritizing the baby's needs.

Giving birth can be challenging. Some moms have an ideal birth plan, and if it doesn't go as planned, it can cause anxiety or even sadness. Understanding this helps us be compassionate and open to the mom sharing her experience.

Some moms wanted a specific birth setup but ended up with something different. They might feel like they didn't have a say in the process, leading to confusion and trauma. Being open, empathetic, and patient is crucial. We allow her to relax, talk about her experience, and assure her that she's doing well.

This chapter connects to the manual's beginning. Our role as intuitive caregivers is to understand the baby's needs and meet the mom where she is. We must put aside our preferences and use tact and wisdom. How we say things matters more than what we say.

Understanding the challenges and emotions mothers may face after childbirth, such as trauma or disappointment, helps us provide compassionate and empathetic care. Allowing them to share their birth stories and supporting them in connecting with their babies is a crucial aspect of our role as infant care specialists. These conversations can be beautiful and enriching to both you and the parents. Our ultimate aim is to be intuitive caregivers, meeting the needs of both the baby and the mother with empathy and wisdom.

19.1 Rubin's Stages of Postpartum

Rubin's Stages of Postpartum refers to a theoretical framework that describes the psychological and physiological adjustment that new mothers experience after childbirth. The stages were first proposed by Dr. Lillian Rubin, a sociologist and psychotherapist, in 1984. According to Rubin, there are four stages of postpartum:

After Glow - Taking-in Stage: This stage occurs in the first few days after birth when the mother focuses on her needs and recovery. She may feel exhausted and overwhelmed; her primary concern is rest, nutrition, and bonding with the baby.

- Mother feels overwhelming relief from late pregnancy and labor discomfort.
- Joy and pride in her newborn.
- Experiences an adrenalin rush and high levels of endorphins.
- The learning curve is very low due to sensory overload.
- Feels and accepts being "taken care of."
- This stage may last 3-5 days.

Caregivers should avoid overloading information or giving lengthy advice; it will not be retained at this stage. Instead, look for "windows of opportunity" to encourage and reinforce appropriate skills.

Coming Back - Taking-hold Stage: This stage usually begins within the first week after birth and can last from a week to several weeks. During this time, the mother becomes more confident and actively cares for her baby. She may be anxious to learn about breastfeeding, managing the baby's sleep schedule, and establishing a routine.

- Mother is beginning to integrate the experience.
- Still feels vulnerable and dependent on caregivers for everyday living needs.
- Starts asking questions about baby and self-care.
- Takes steps toward self-care and appearance.
- Feels fatigued and frustrated.
- The caregiver should attend to the physical needs of the mother and baby.

Continue to encourage and reassure her. You are there to help meet her and the baby's needs. Let her know she is doing well and what she is experiencing is normal. This stage is the most difficult due to extreme hormonal changes. The body realizes it does not have the placenta, and pregnancy hormones decline and are replaced by lactation hormones.

"I can do this" - Letting-go Stage: This stage usually occurs within the first month after birth and involves the mother coming to terms with the reality of motherhood. She may experience a range of emotions, including sadness, anxiety, and guilt, as she adjusts to the demands of caring for a newborn.

- Mother is hopefully empowered by the experience and beginning to master infant care and feeding tasks.
- Fatigued but adapting to schedule.
- Takes an interest in hygiene and personal appearance.
- May be processing any disappointments in experience or appearance.
- Begins to see herself as a parent and develops a stronger bond with her baby.
- Feels a sense of pride in her ability to care for her child
- Begins to develop a vision of the parent she wants to be.

It's important to note that these stages are not always linear, and not every mother will experience them similarly. However, understanding these stages can help new mothers and their partners anticipate and prepare for the challenges and changes of becoming a parent.

19.2 Postpartum Depression

After the baby's birth, the mother experiences many changes in her body. Hormones fluctuate, and she may cry easily, feel depressed, have a loss of appetite, struggle to concentrate, and find it challenging to sleep. These symptoms are typical and may last up to ten days. Improvement typically occurs.

However, some women may develop postpartum depression (PPD), a treatable disease, using drugs, therapy, and networking with other mothers. PPD is estimated to affect up to 15% of women who have recently given birth, although the exact prevalence varies depending on the population studied.

PPD typically develops within the first few months after delivery, but it can occur at any time during the first year postpartum. Symptoms of PPD can include:

- Persistent sadness or hopelessness
- Loss of interest in activities they used to enjoy
- Difficulty sleeping or sleeping too much
- Fatigue or lack of energy
- Changes in appetite or weight
- Anxiety or irritability
- Difficulty concentrating or making decisions
- Thoughts of harming themselves or their baby
- Feelings of loss
- Impatience, bouts of crying, mood swings
- Feeling worthless or hopeless
- Feeling like life is not worth living

The exact causes of PPD are not fully understood, but researchers believe that a combination of physical, emotional, and social factors can contribute to its development. Hormonal changes that occur during and after pregnancy are thought to play a role, as well as sleep deprivation, lack of social support, and a history of depression or other mental health issues.

Postpartum depression is more likely if the woman had previous PPD, depression not related to pregnancy, a family history of mental illness, severe premenstrual syndrome (PMS), a difficult marriage, stressful life events, or a birth that did not go as planned.

Women with PPD should seek help from a mental health professional as soon as possible, as prompt treatment can improve outcomes for both the mother and the baby. In addition to professional therapy, self-care strategies such as exercise, healthy eating, and getting enough sleep can also help manage symptoms of PPD.

If unsure whether it's the blues or PPD, encourage the mother to call a doctor or professional. If she can't make the call, have her talk to a partner, parent, sibling, or friend to arrange help. If she can't talk about it, hand this page to someone close to her. Treatment is available, even if she is breastfeeding.

Postnatal Depression Scale

About 50% of women with Postpartum Depression are undiagnosed. The following scale can be used in the third trimester to help identify women at risk for postpartum depression. The scale can also be used after birth.

PPD Self-Assessment Questionnaire

(Taken from Postpartum Education for Parents)

The scale is a self-reporting screening tool. Rate each question (yes, no, or sometimes) based on how the mother felt in the last seven days, not just that day. She might want to discuss these results with a qualified therapist if warranted.

- I have been able to laugh and see the funny side of things.
- I have looked forward with enjoyment to things.
- I have blamed myself unnecessarily when things go wrong.
- I have been anxious or worried for no good reason.
- I have felt scared or panicky for no good reason.
- Things have been getting on top of me.
- I have been so unhappy that I have had difficulty sleeping.
- I have felt sad or miserable.
- I have been so unhappy that I have been crying.
- The thought of harming myself has occurred to me.

How Can You Help Mom Get Rid Of The Blues?

- Encourage her to join a support group.
- Protect her from unwanted visitors.
- Tell Dad what he can do to help.

- Encourage her to get some sleep.
- Have her talk about her feelings.
- Get help from others.
- Attend to the baby for her.
- Be patient and encourage her.

Appendex

Taxes

As a Newborn Care Specialist, you will work as an Independent Contractor (check on whether to include info about Employee versus IC).

Medicine Consent Form

(SAMPLE) feel free to use this form

__________________________ (name of parent) give permission for ___ (Newborn Care Specialist) to give my child _______________ (Name of the child) the following medication ___________________________for _____________ (reason) for taking medication).

The dosage for this medication is___________________(dosage) to be given every _______ (frequency).

The last dose was administered today at:___________ Side effects to watch out for may include: (List all of the possible side effects):

This medicine was prescribed by: ____________________________ (Name of Doctor)

Signature of Parent__________________________ Date________ _

About Joy

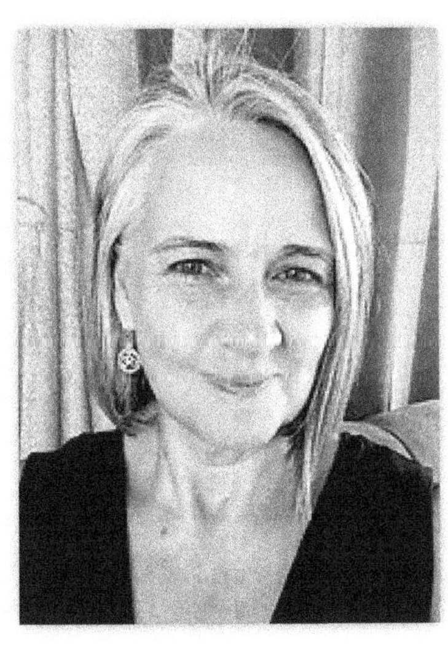

I'm Joy Bostrom, Founder of the JOY of Sleep. I am a postpartum doula with over 10 years of experience in single-baby and twin care, and I'm also a mother of two young men. I was born in England to American parents and I was raised in Mexico from age 3-17. I'm fluent in both English and Spanish. As an adult, I have lived all over the United States and in Costa Rica. Before becoming a doula, I worked in the medical field as a Medical Assistant.

I've had a love for babies and a passion for helping from a very young age and I feel privileged to work in something I'm passionate about! Through my years of work and multi-cultural knowledge, I've found many helpful strategies, tools, and techniques to help babies sleep better and longer.

As I've grown alongside the JOY of Sleep, I've come to realize that more parents are searching for compassionate infant care and family support. Now, the Joy of Sleep team is expanding from one person (me) to an amazing team of women with the same shared vision, utilizing the JOY of Sleep method to help parents and infants all over the world.

We are excited to share with you the JOY of Sleep method and help make caring for your newborn a fun and memorable experience.

www.ingramcontent.com/pod-product-compliance
Ingram Content Group UK Ltd.
Pitfield, Milton Keynes, MK11 3LW, UK
UKHW062000290726
14090UKWH00021B/1301

9 798869 151216